How to use
this Food Diary ...

Track what matters to you: sugar, caffeine, omega-3 etc.

Learn where & when you eat the right and wrong foods, to help correct bad habits.

Find your Base Calorie Requirement, and calories burnt during different activities, in the tables at the back of the book.

Learn your own personal keys to success with a daily review and calorie balance calculation.

Food & Drink

Time & Place	Item	Amount	Protein	Fat	Carbs	Iron	Cals
Home, 7:15	Muesli + milk	1x bowl	7g	8g	28g	1.5mg	211
	Banana		1g	0.5g	23g	0.3mg	90
Work 10:45	Small decaf latte		6g	4g	9g		98
Lunch with Jane 1:10	Chicken & Avocado Sub		27g	14g	56g	2.5mg	468
	Sparkling water						0!
On way home from work	Carrot cake	x1 piece	6g	15g	37g	1.5mg	295
Early evening meal (5pm) with kids	Salmon Fish Cakes	x3	17g	3g	23g	1mg	179
	+ Salad & rice		5g	11g	31g	1mg	239
	Tap water						
9pm with John	Hummus & cucumber + Pitta	x2 pittas	13g	11g	40g	3mg	311
	1 x glass red wine				3g	find out!	85
							1976

Exercise

Time & Place	Type & Intensity	Alone / with Company?	Duration	Cals
Work	Standing up		2 hrs	275
	Walked back from work moderate pace	alone	20 mins	102
	Base Calorie Requirement			1800
				2177

Review: Tomorrow take a healthy snack and a drink! for the way home from work.

-210 Balance

Day 2

10/1

Sleep — Poor-Up in night with Jack

Drink enough each day.

Supplements

Medication

Tick off your 5 portions of fruit & veg each day to make sure you don't miss one.

Allergies   Stress   Energy

Pinpoint any triggers of allergies.

Daily Goal

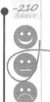

Finish work in time to walk home ✗ ✓

Set yourself small, achieveable targets with the 'daily goal'

Review and plan your daily goals within the Personal Statistics Tracker at the back of the book.

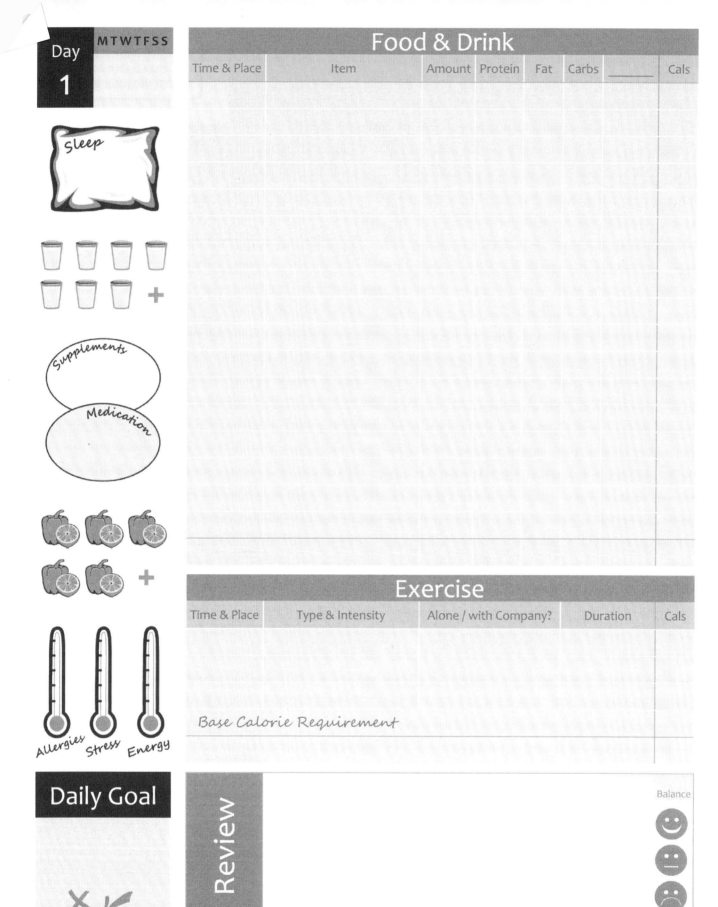

Day 1

MTWTFSS

Sleep

Supplements

Medication

Allergies Stress Energy

Daily Goal

X ✔

Food & Drink

Time & Place	Item	Amount	Protein	Fat	Carbs	_____	Cals

Exercise

Time & Place	Type & Intensity	Alone / with Company?	Duration	Cals

Base Calorie Requirement

Review

Balance

😊

😐

☹️

Food & Drink

Time & Place	Item	Amount	Protein	Fat	Carbs		Cals

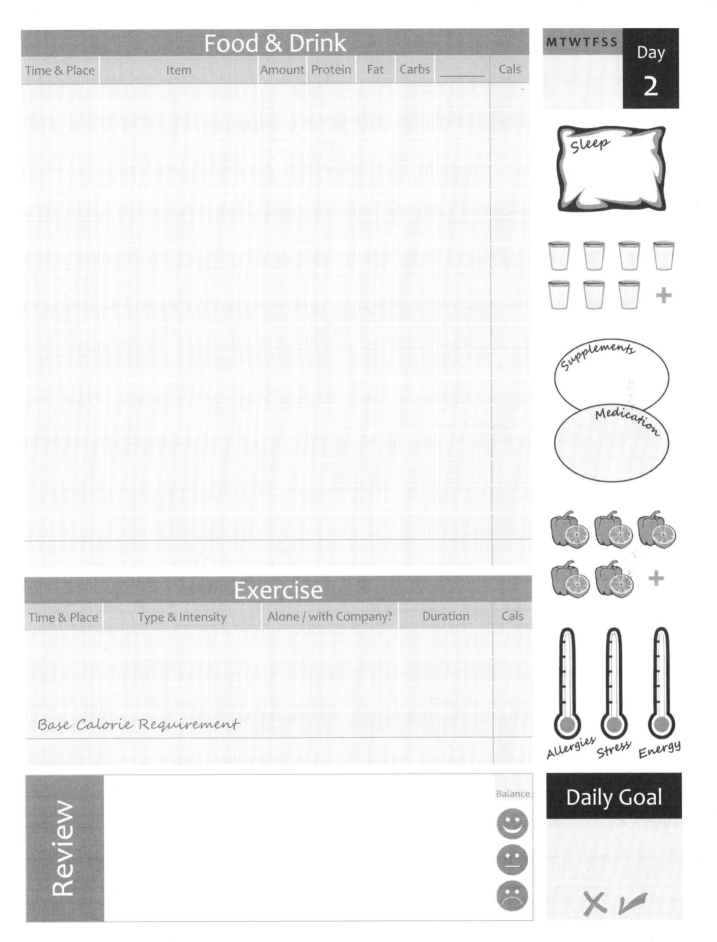

MTWTFSS — Day 2

Sleep

Supplements

Medication

Exercise

Time & Place	Type & Intensity	Alone / with Company?	Duration	Cals
Base Calorie Requirement				

Allergies   Stress   Energy

Review

Balance

Daily Goal

X ✔

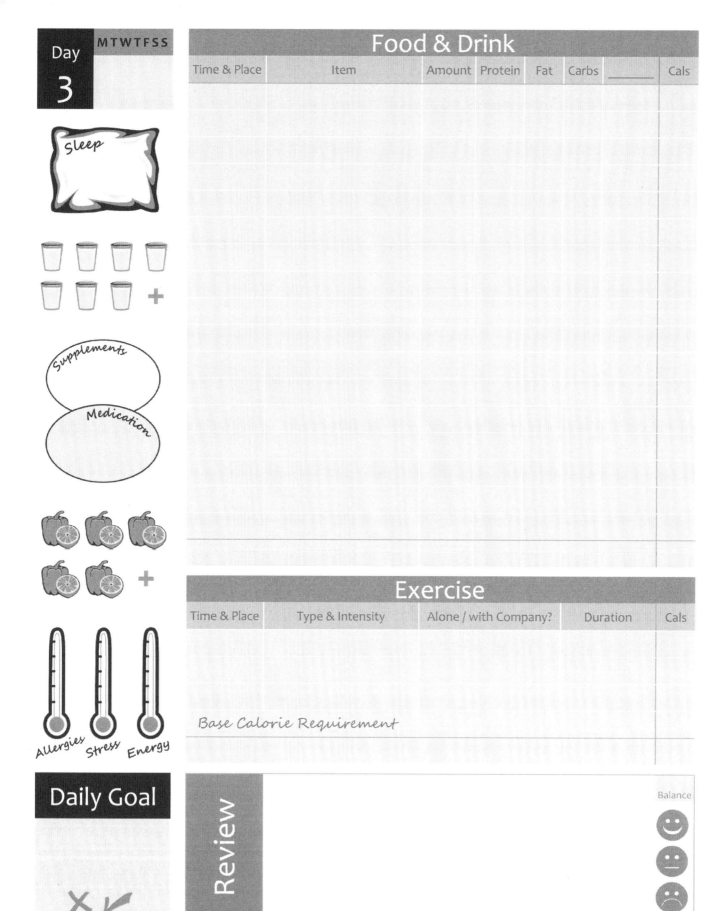

Day 3 M T W T F S S

Sleep

Supplements

Medication

Allergies Stress Energy

Daily Goal

X ✔

Food & Drink

Time & Place	Item	Amount	Protein	Fat	Carbs	_____	Cals

Exercise

Time & Place	Type & Intensity	Alone / with Company?	Duration	Cals
Base Calorie Requirement				

Review

Balance

Food & Drink

Time & Place	Item	Amount	Protein	Fat	Carbs	_____	Cals

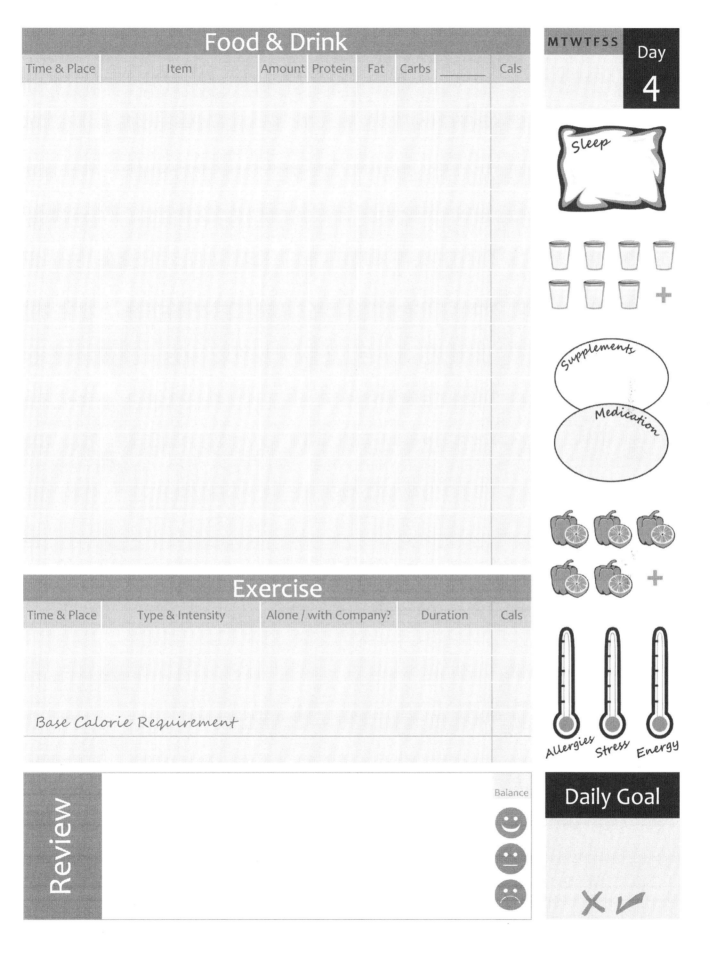

MTWTFSS

Day 4

Sleep

Supplements

Medication

+

+

Allergies Stress Energy

Exercise

Time & Place	Type & Intensity	Alone / with Company?	Duration	Cals
Base Calorie Requirement				

Review

Balance

Daily Goal

X ✔

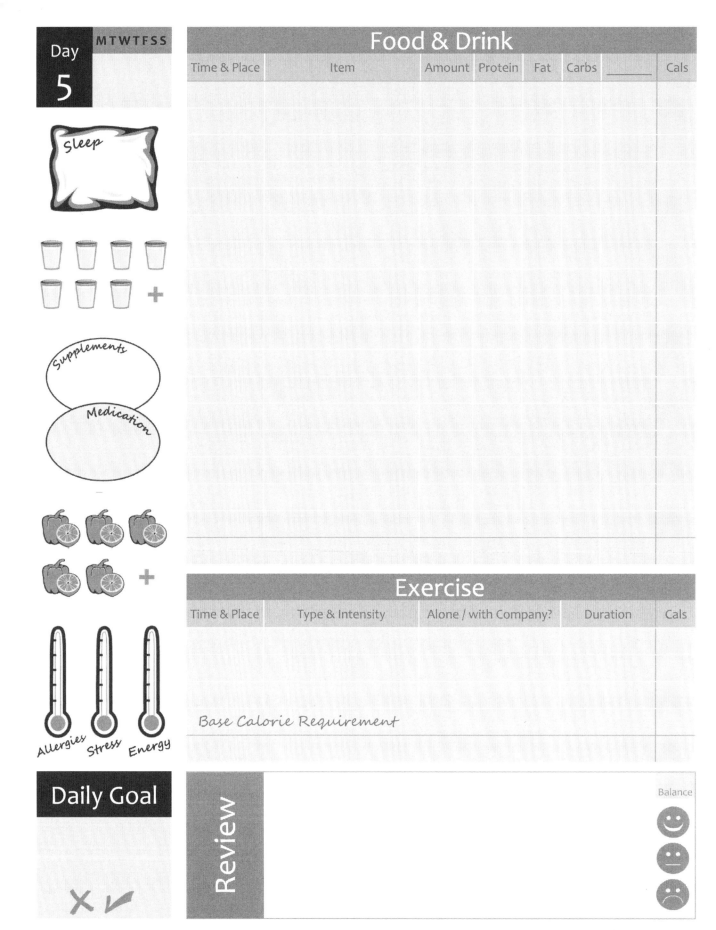

Day 5
MTWTFSS

Sleep

Supplements

Medication

Allergies Stress Energy

Daily Goal
X ✔

Food & Drink

Time & Place	Item	Amount	Protein	Fat	Carbs	____	Cals

Exercise

Time & Place	Type & Intensity	Alone / with Company?	Duration	Cals
Base Calorie Requirement				

Review

Balance

Food & Drink

Time & Place	Item	Amount	Protein	Fat	Carbs	_____	Cals

Exercise

Time & Place	Type & Intensity	Alone / with Company?	Duration	Cals
Base Calorie Requirement				

Review

Balance

Daily Goal

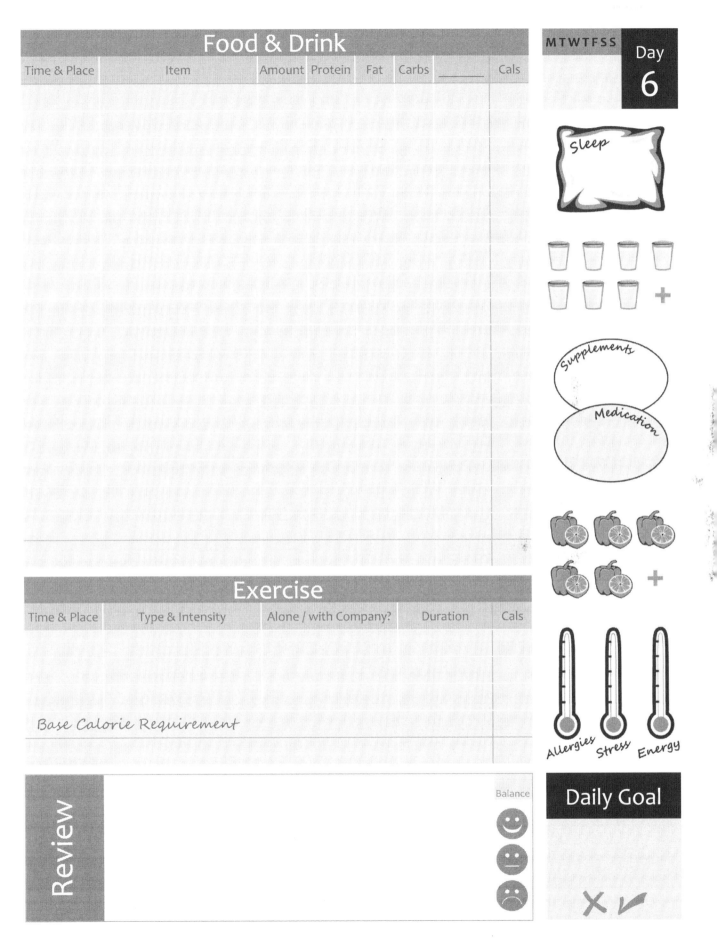

Sleep

Supplements

Medication

Allergies   Stress   Energy

X ✔

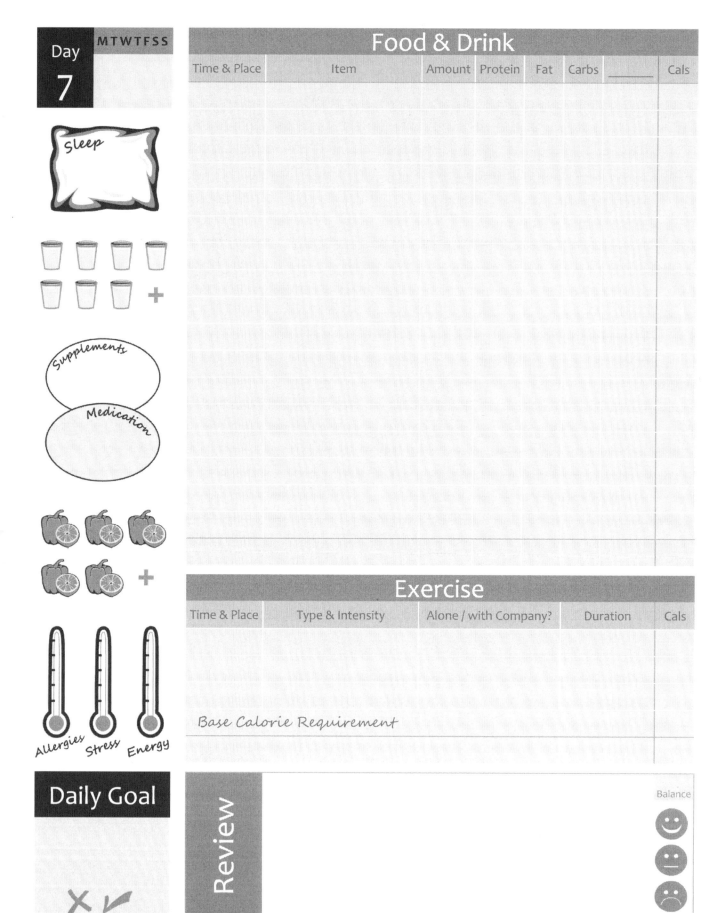

Day 7 — MTWTFSS

Sleep

Supplements

Medication

Allergies   Stress   Energy

Daily Goal
X ✔

Food & Drink

Time & Place	Item	Amount	Protein	Fat	Carbs	_____	Cals

Exercise

Time & Place	Type & Intensity	Alone / with Company?	Duration	Cals
Base Calorie Requirement				

Review

Balance

Food & Drink

Time & Place	Item	Amount	Protein	Fat	Carbs	_____	Cals

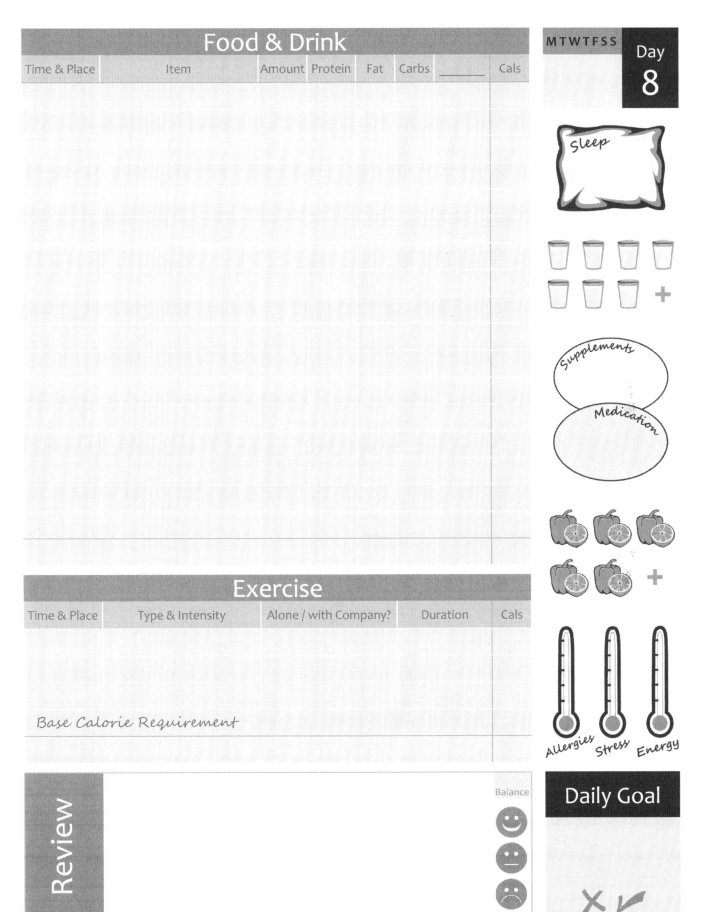

Sleep

Supplements

Medication

Exercise

Time & Place	Type & Intensity	Alone / with Company?	Duration	Cals

Base Calorie Requirement

Allergies Stress Energy

Review

Balance

Daily Goal

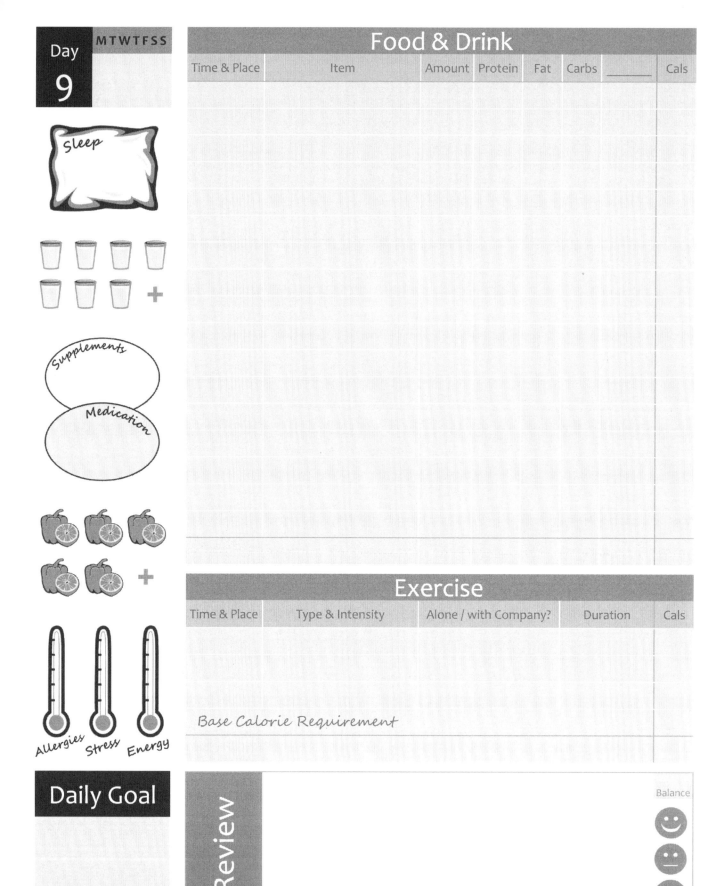

Day 9

MTWTFSS

Sleep

Supplements

Medication

Allergies   Stress   Energy

Daily Goal

X ✔

Food & Drink

Time & Place	Item	Amount	Protein	Fat	Carbs		Cals

Exercise

Time & Place	Type & Intensity	Alone / with Company?	Duration	Cals
Base Calorie Requirement				

Review

Balance

Food & Drink

Time & Place	Item	Amount	Protein	Fat	Carbs		Cals

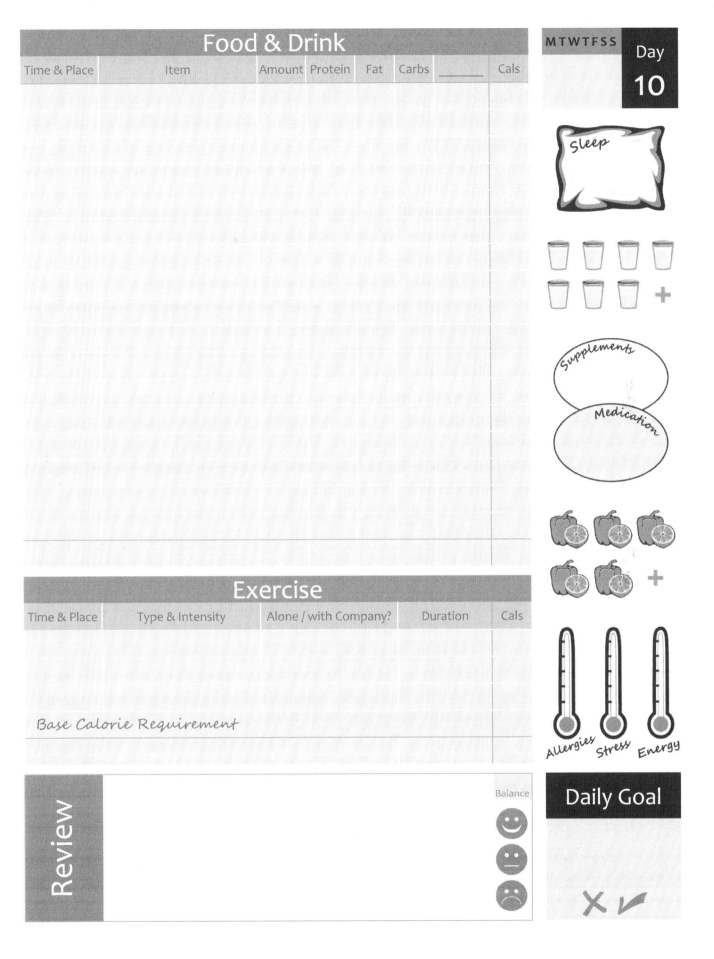

Sleep

Supplements

Medication

Exercise

Time & Place	Type & Intensity	Alone / with Company?	Duration	Cals
Base Calorie Requirement				

Allergies   Stress   Energy

Review

Balance

Daily Goal

X ✔

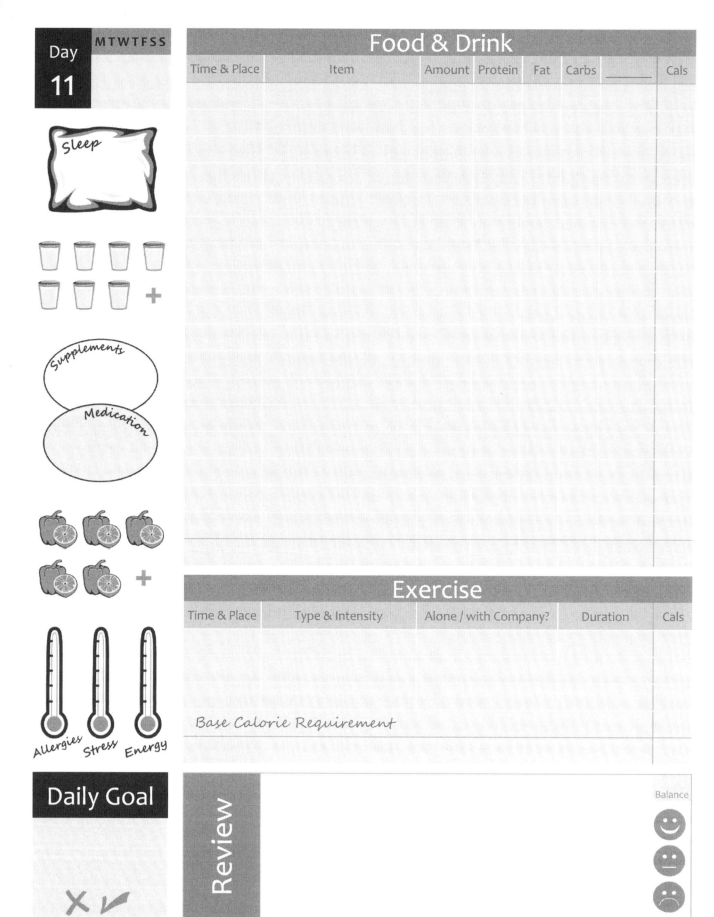

Day 11

MTWTFSS

Sleep

Supplements

Medication

Allergies   Stress   Energy

Daily Goal

X ✔

Food & Drink

Time & Place	Item	Amount	Protein	Fat	Carbs	_____	Cals

Exercise

Time & Place	Type & Intensity	Alone / with Company?	Duration	Cals
Base Calorie Requirement				

Review

Balance

Food & Drink

Time & Place	Item	Amount	Protein	Fat	Carbs	_____	Cals

Day 12

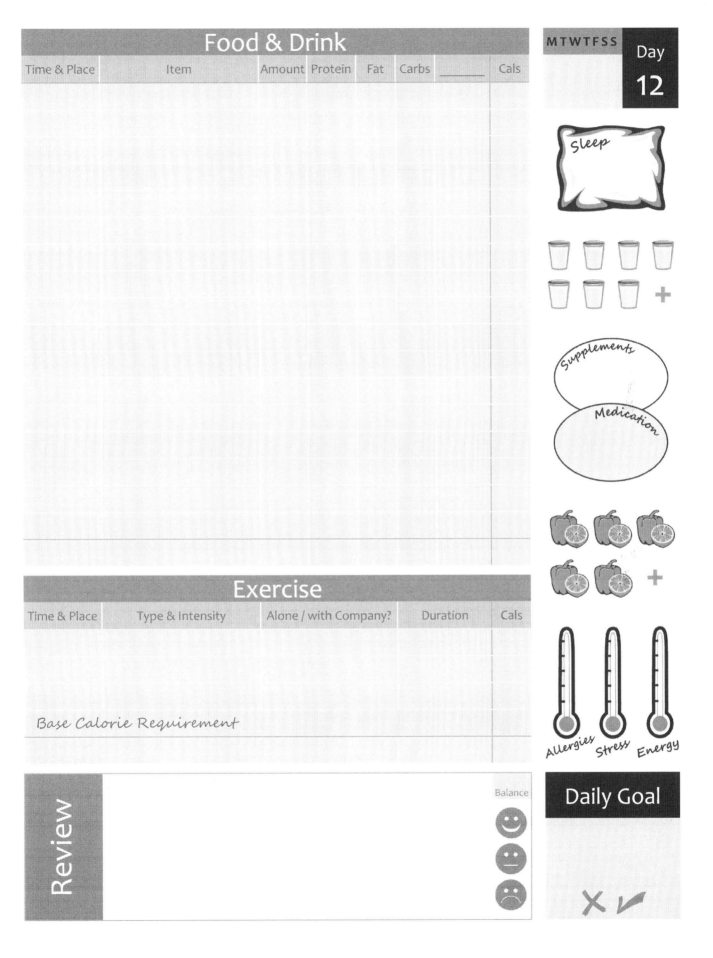

Sleep

Supplements

Medication

Exercise

Time & Place	Type & Intensity	Alone / with Company?	Duration	Cals
Base Calorie Requirement				

Allergies   Stress   Energy

Review

Balance

Daily Goal

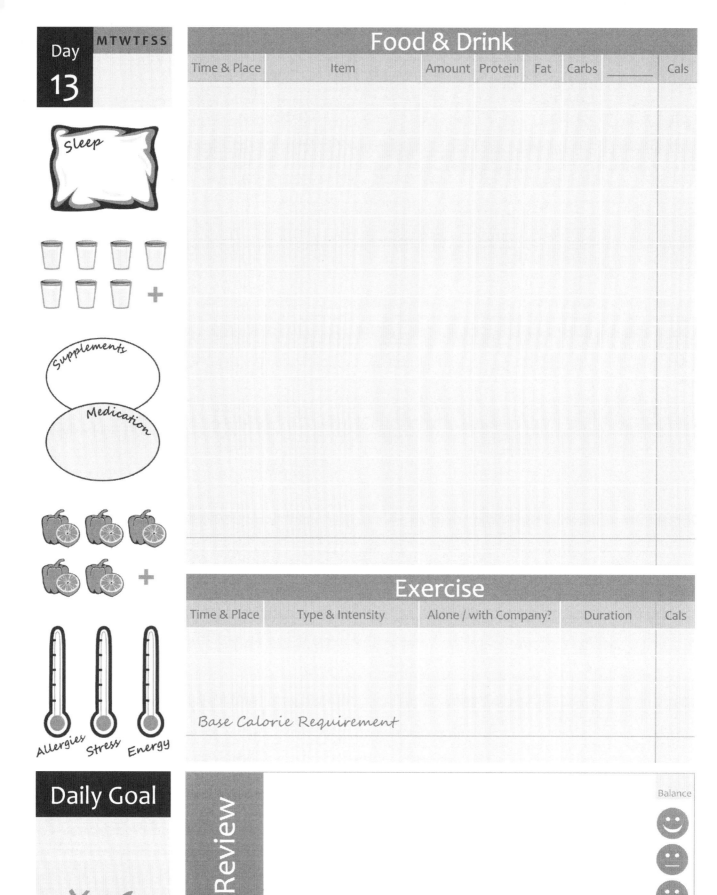

Day 13 MTWTFSS

Sleep

Supplements

Medication

Allergies Stress Energy

Daily Goal

X ✔

Food & Drink

Time & Place	Item	Amount	Protein	Fat	Carbs	_____	Cals

Exercise

Time & Place	Type & Intensity	Alone / with Company?	Duration	Cals

Base Calorie Requirement

Review

Balance

Food & Drink

Time & Place	Item	Amount	Protein	Fat	Carbs	_____	Cals

Sleep

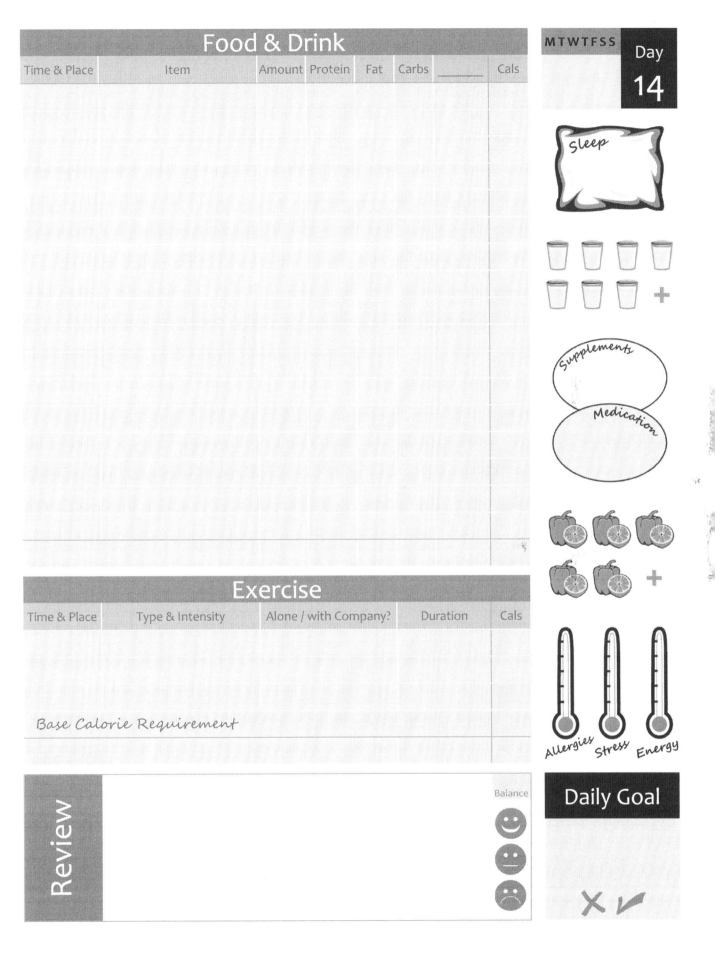

Supplements

Medication

Exercise

Time & Place	Type & Intensity	Alone / with Company?	Duration	Cals
Base Calorie Requirement				

Allergies Stress Energy

Review

Balance

Daily Goal

X ✔

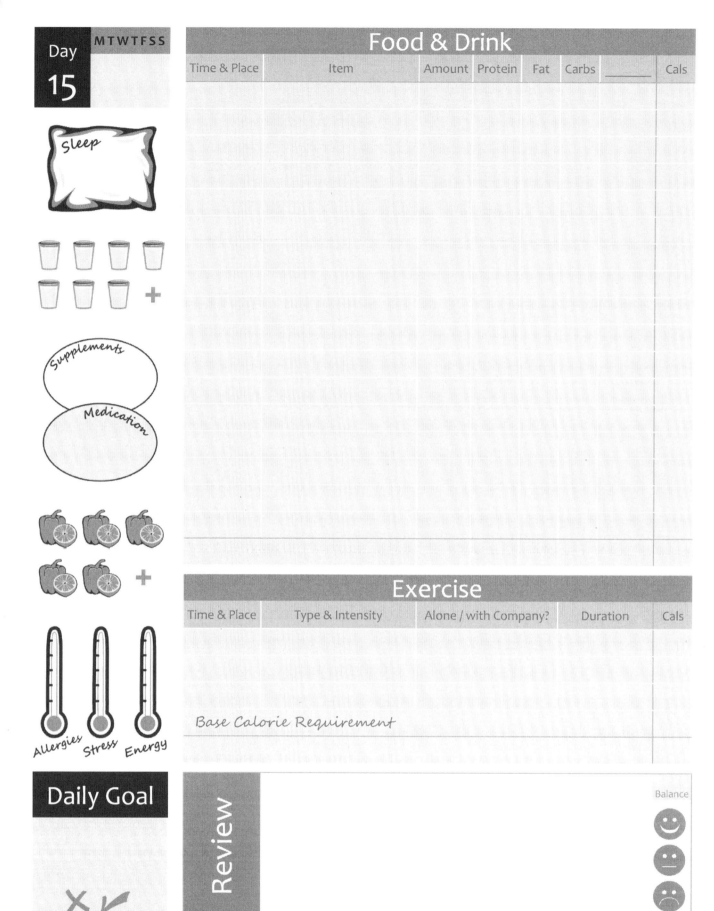

Day 15

MTWTFSS

Sleep

Supplements

Medication

Allergies Stress Energy

Daily Goal

X ✔

Food & Drink

Time & Place	Item	Amount	Protein	Fat	Carbs	_____	Cals

Exercise

Time & Place	Type & Intensity	Alone / with Company?	Duration	Cals
Base Calorie Requirement				

Review

Balance

☺
😐
☹

Food & Drink

Time & Place	Item	Amount	Protein	Fat	Carbs	_____	Cals

Exercise

Time & Place	Type & Intensity	Alone / with Company?	Duration	Cals
Base Calorie Requirement				

Review

Balance

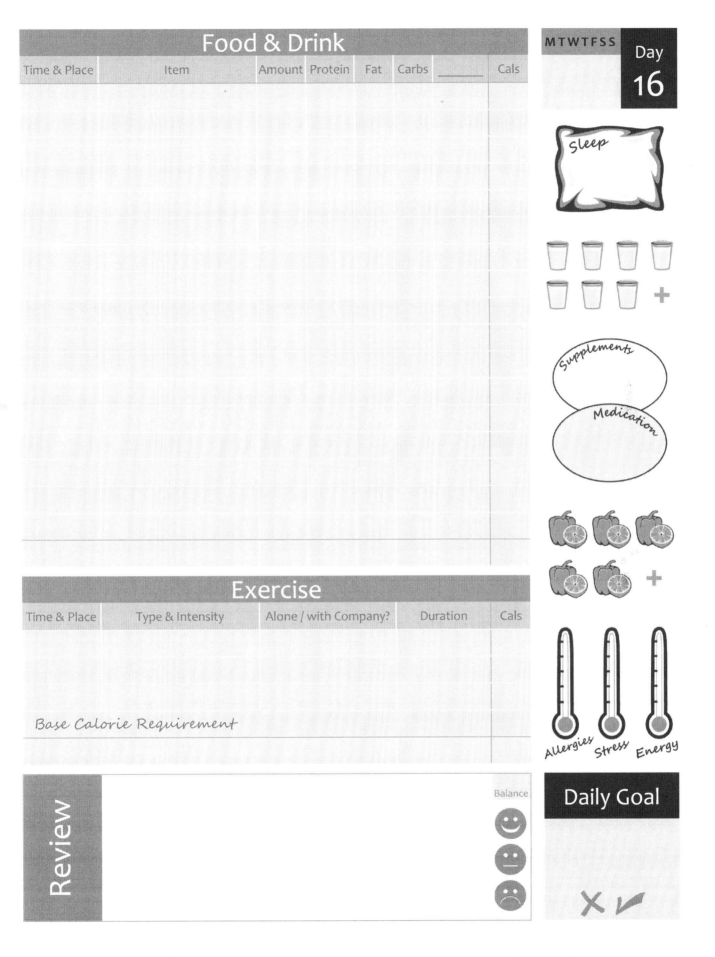

Sleep

Supplements

Medication

Allergies Stress Energy

Daily Goal

X ✔

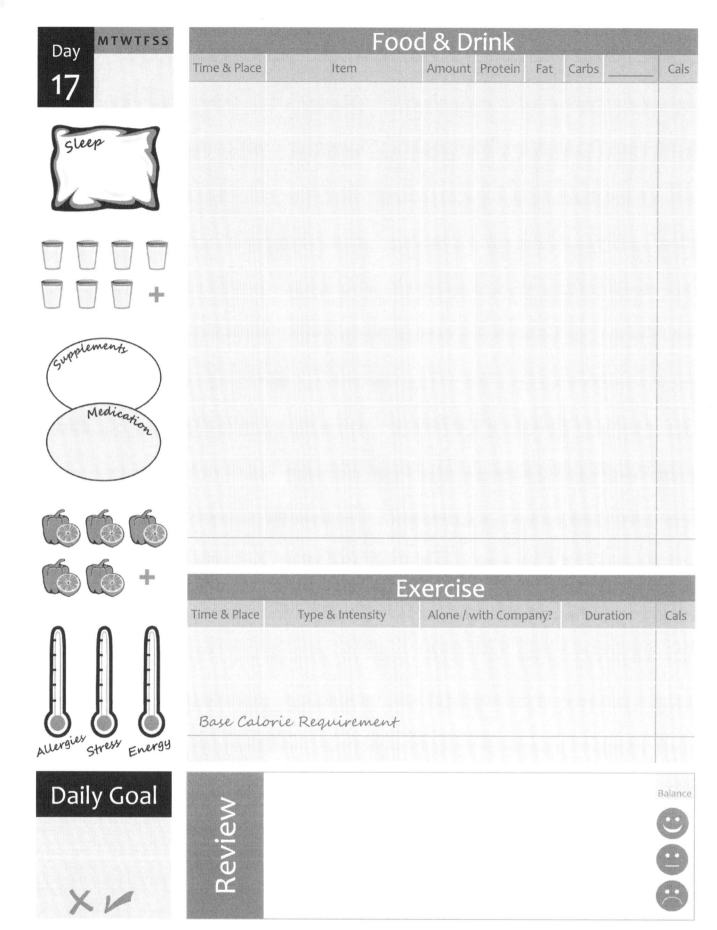

Day 17

MTWTFSS

Sleep

Supplements

Medication

Allergies Stress Energy

Daily Goal

X ✔

Food & Drink

Time & Place	Item	Amount	Protein	Fat	Carbs		Cals

Exercise

Time & Place	Type & Intensity	Alone / with Company?	Duration	Cals
Base Calorie Requirement				

Review

Balance

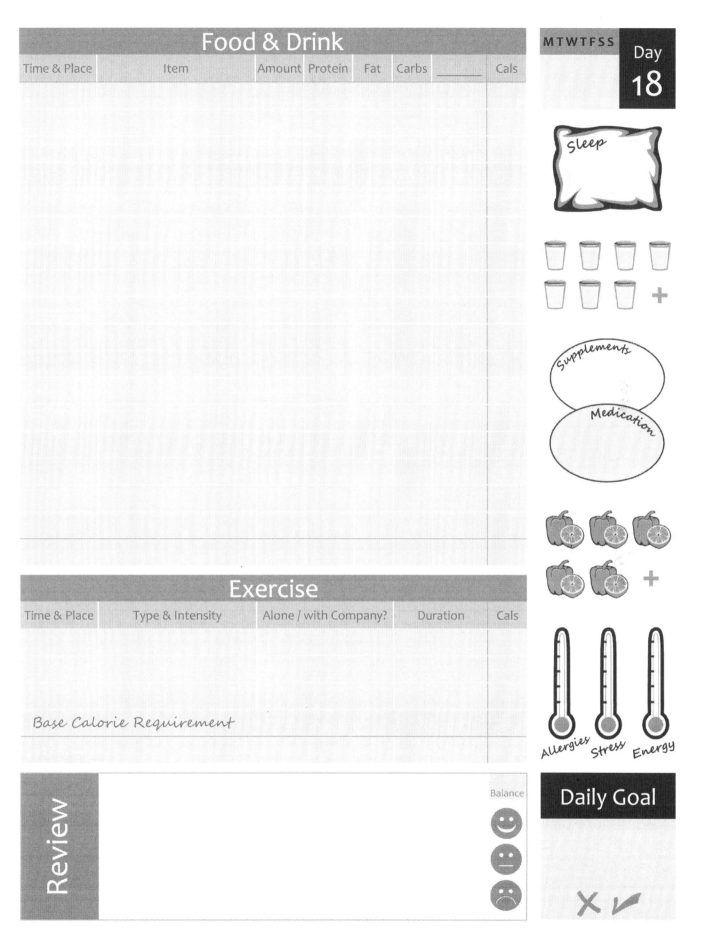

Food & Drink

Time & Place	Item	Amount	Protein	Fat	Carbs	_____	Cals

Sleep

Supplements

Medication

Exercise

Time & Place	Type & Intensity	Alone / with Company?	Duration	Cals
Base Calorie Requirement				

Allergies   Stress   Energy

Review

Balance

Daily Goal

X ✔

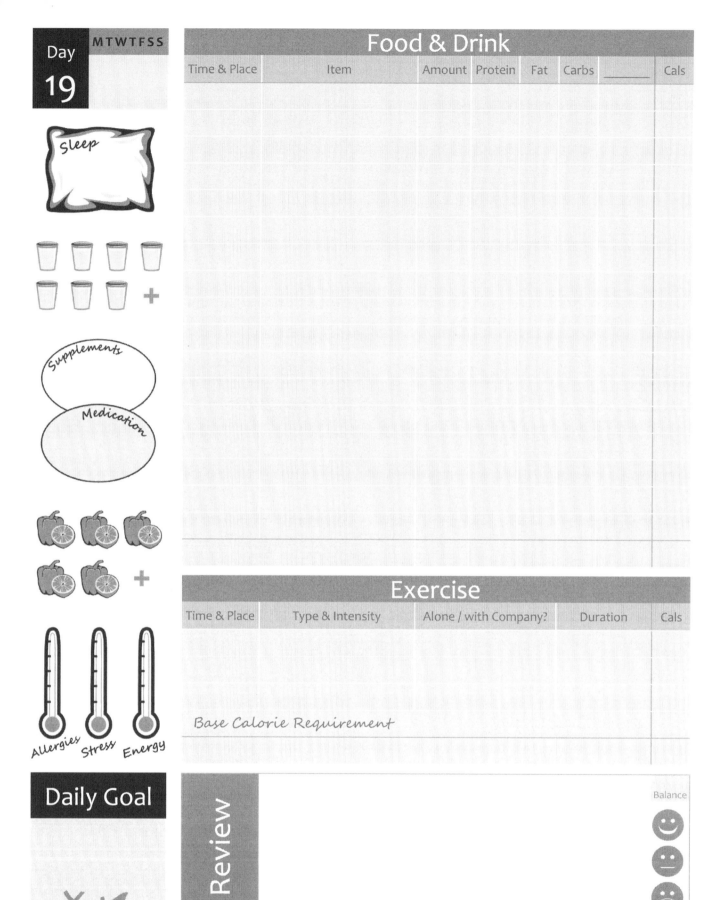

Sleep

Supplements

Medication

Allergies   Stress   Energy

Daily Goal

✗ ✔

Food & Drink

Time & Place	Item	Amount	Protein	Fat	Carbs		Cals

Exercise

Time & Place	Type & Intensity	Alone / with Company?	Duration	Cals
Base Calorie Requirement				

Review

Balance

Food & Drink

Time & Place	Item	Amount	Protein	Fat	Carbs	_____	Cals

Sleep

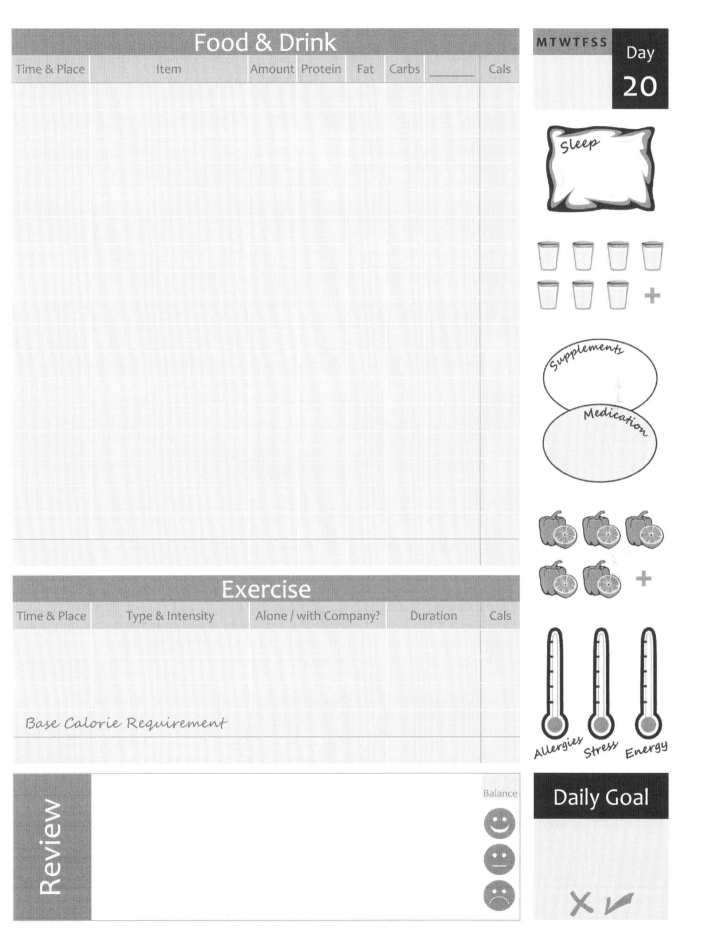

Supplements

Medication

Exercise

Time & Place	Type & Intensity	Alone / with Company?	Duration	Cals
Base Calorie Requirement				

Allergies Stress Energy

Review

Balance

Daily Goal

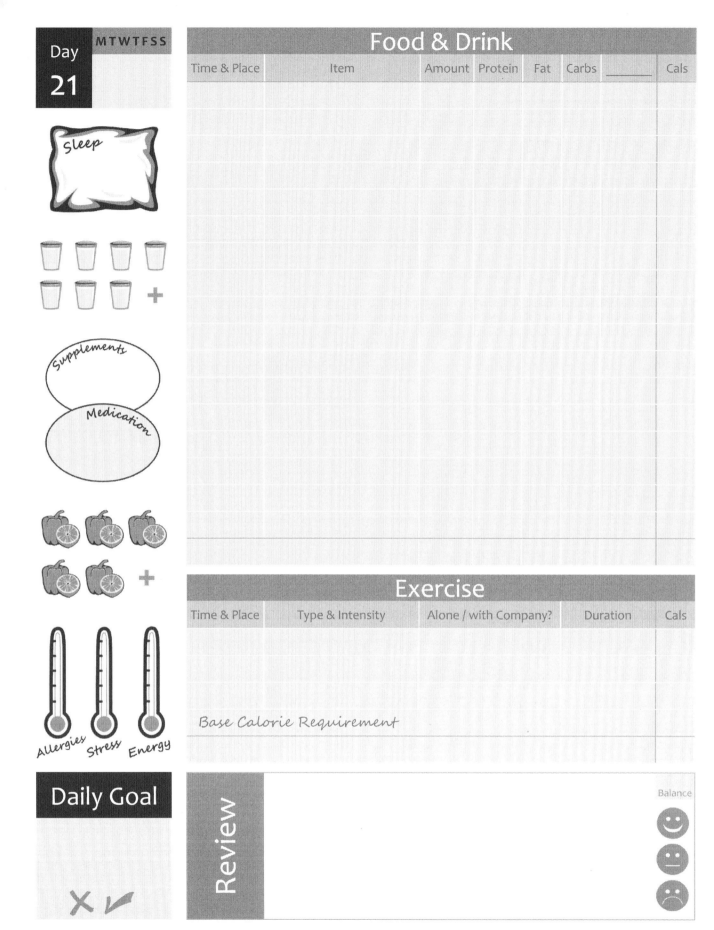

Day 21

MTWTFSS

Sleep

Supplements

Medication

Allergies Stress Energy

Daily Goal

X ✔

Food & Drink

Time & Place	Item	Amount	Protein	Fat	Carbs		Cals

Exercise

Time & Place	Type & Intensity	Alone / with Company?	Duration	Cals

Base Calorie Requirement

Review

Balance

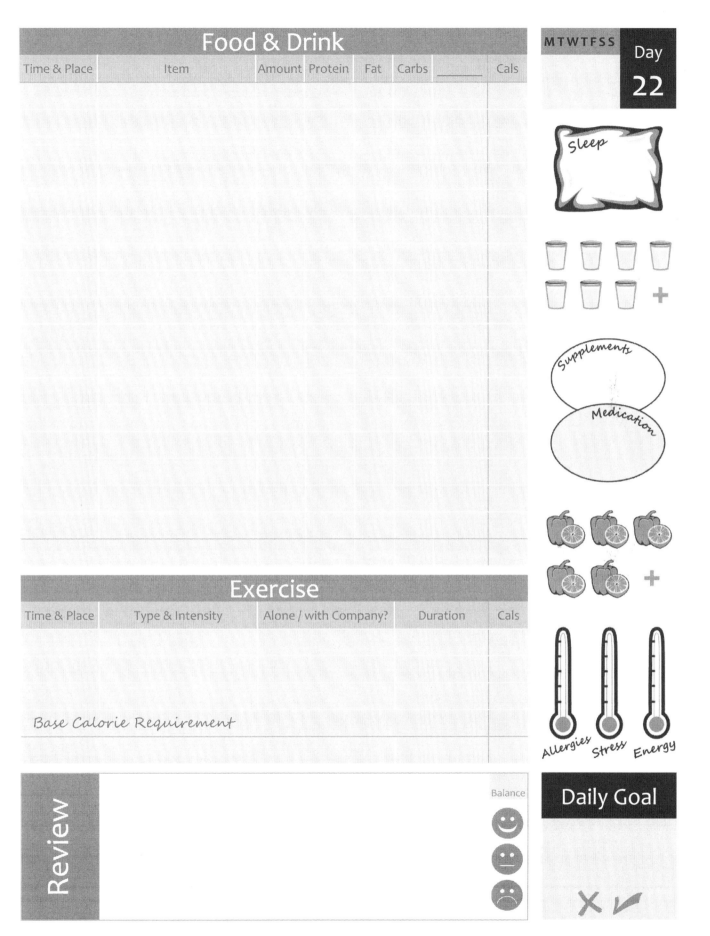

Food & Drink

Time & Place	Item	Amount	Protein	Fat	Carbs	_____	Cals

MTWTFSS

Day 22

Sleep

Supplements

Medication

Allergies   Stress   Energy

Exercise

Time & Place	Type & Intensity	Alone / with Company?	Duration	Cals

Base Calorie Requirement

Review

Balance

Daily Goal

X ✔

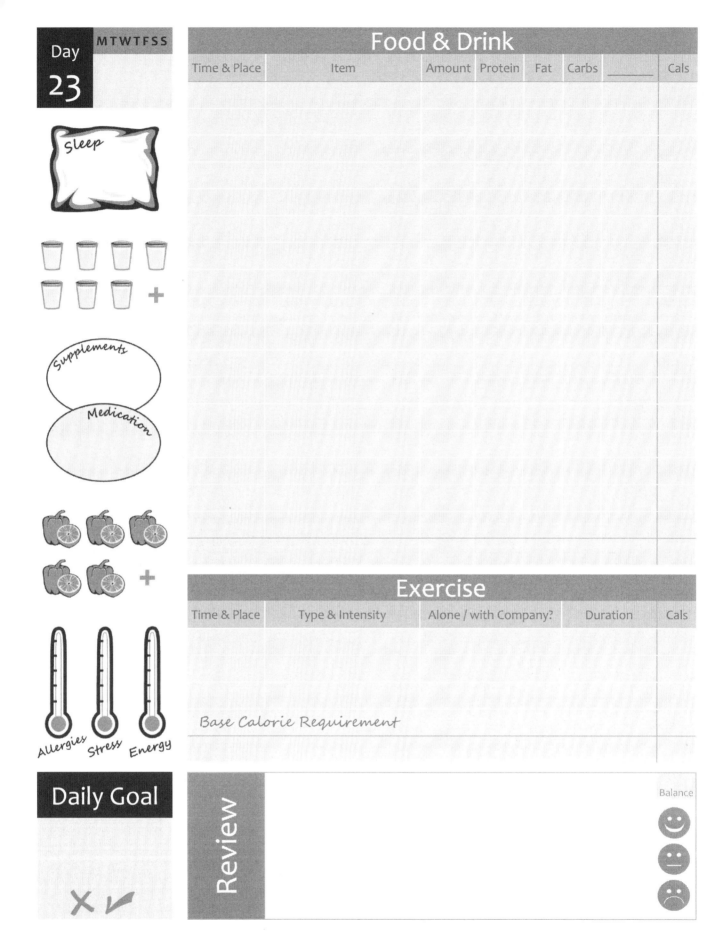

Day
23

MTWTFSS

Sleep

Supplements

Medication

Allergies Stress Energy

Daily Goal

X ✔

Food & Drink

Time & Place	Item	Amount	Protein	Fat	Carbs	_____	Cals

Exercise

Time & Place	Type & Intensity	Alone / with Company?	Duration	Cals

Base Calorie Requirement

Review

Balance

Food & Drink

Time & Place	Item	Amount	Protein	Fat	Carbs	_____	Cals

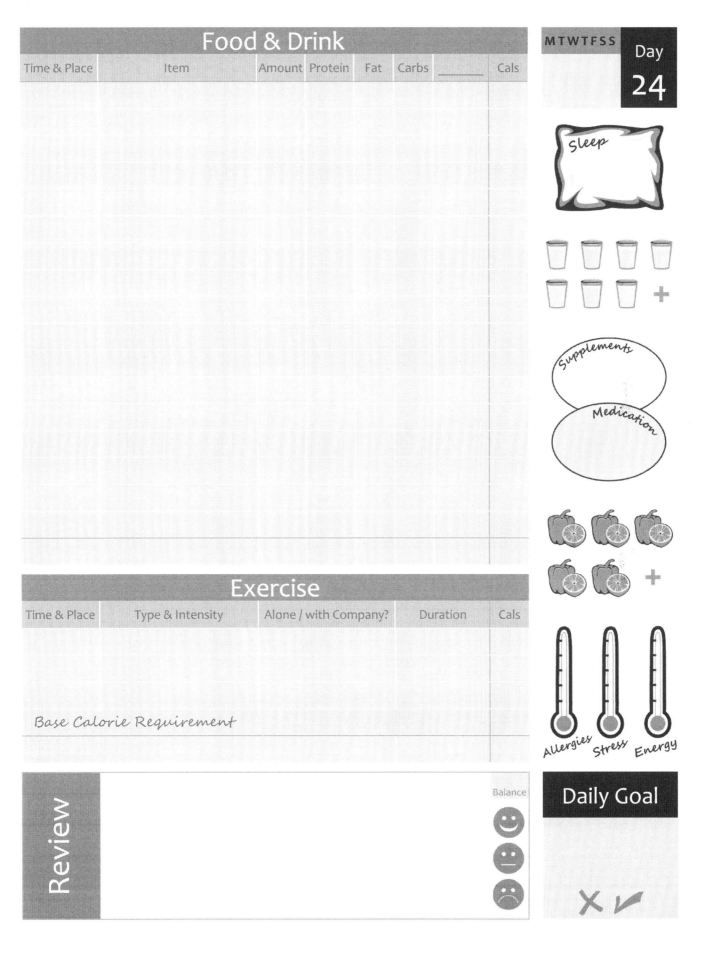

Sleep

Supplements

Medication

Exercise

Time & Place	Type & Intensity	Alone / with Company?	Duration	Cals
Base Calorie Requirement				

Allergies   Stress   Energy

Review

Balance

Daily Goal

X ✔

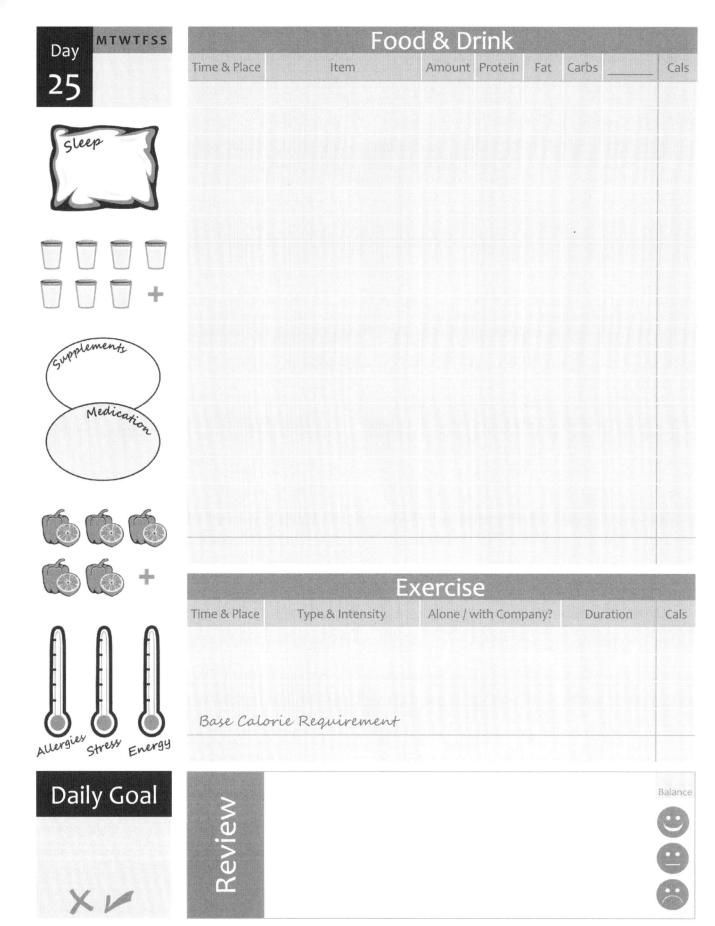

Day 25

MTWTFSS

Sleep

Supplements

Medication

Allergies Stress Energy

Daily Goal

X ✔

Food & Drink

Time & Place	Item	Amount	Protein	Fat	Carbs	_____	Cals

Exercise

Time & Place	Type & Intensity	Alone / with Company?	Duration	Cals

Base Calorie Requirement

Review

Balance

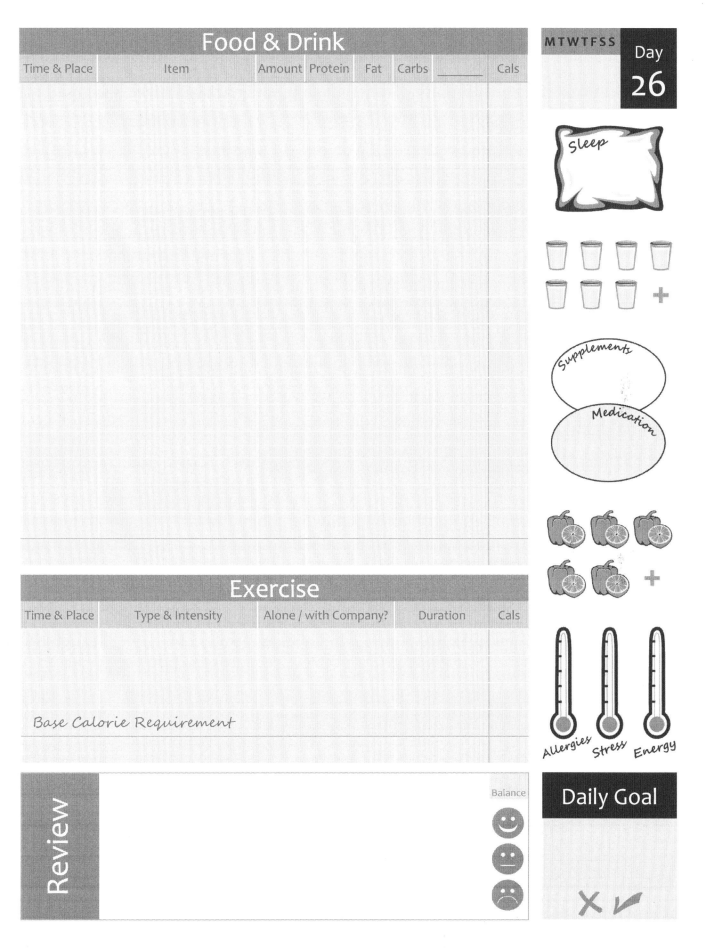

Food & Drink

Time & Place	Item	Amount	Protein	Fat	Carbs	_____	Cals

Sleep

Supplements

Medication

Exercise

Time & Place	Type & Intensity	Alone / with Company?	Duration	Cals
Base Calorie Requirement				

Allergies Stress Energy

Review

Balance

Daily Goal

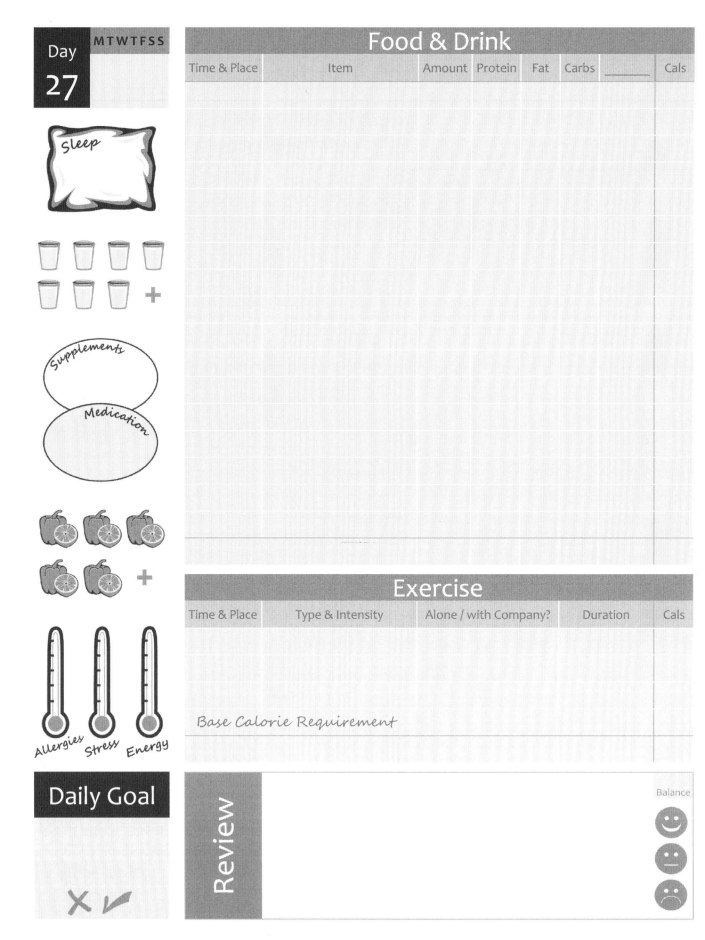

Day
27

MTWTFSS

Sleep

Supplements

Medication

Allergies   Stress   Energy

Daily Goal

✗ ✓

Food & Drink

Time & Place	Item	Amount	Protein	Fat	Carbs	_____	Cals

Exercise

Time & Place	Type & Intensity	Alone / with Company?	Duration	Cals
Base Calorie Requirement				

Review

Balance

☺
😐
☹

Food & Drink

Time & Place	Item	Amount	Protein	Fat	Carbs	_____	Cals

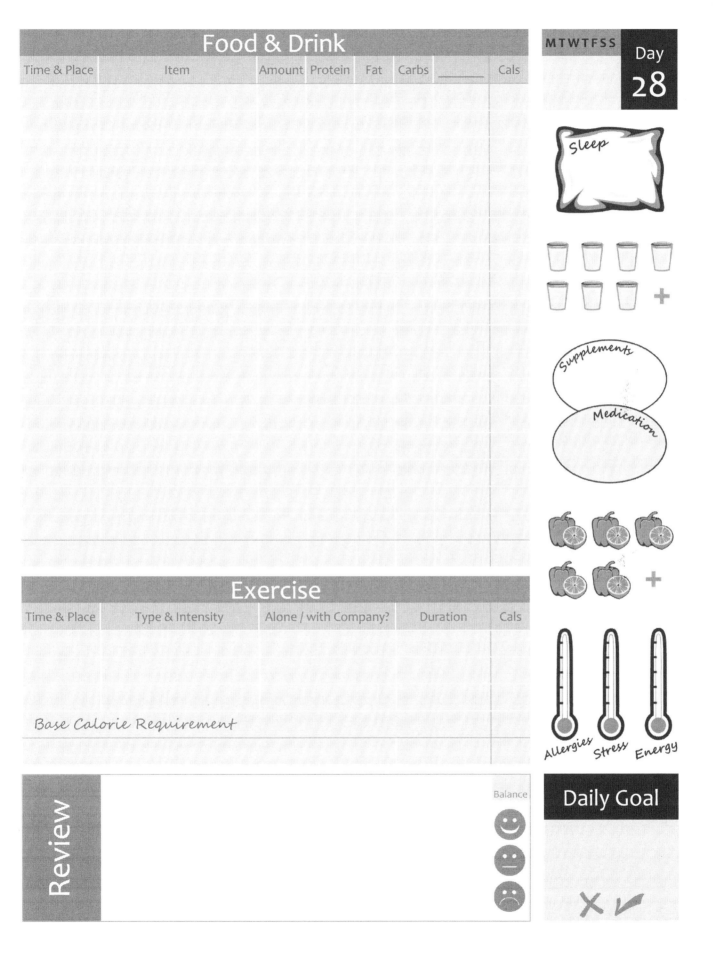

Sleep

Supplements

Medication

Exercise

Time & Place	Type & Intensity	Alone / with Company?	Duration	Cals
Base Calorie Requirement				

Allergies   Stress   Energy

Review

Balance

Daily Goal

X ✔

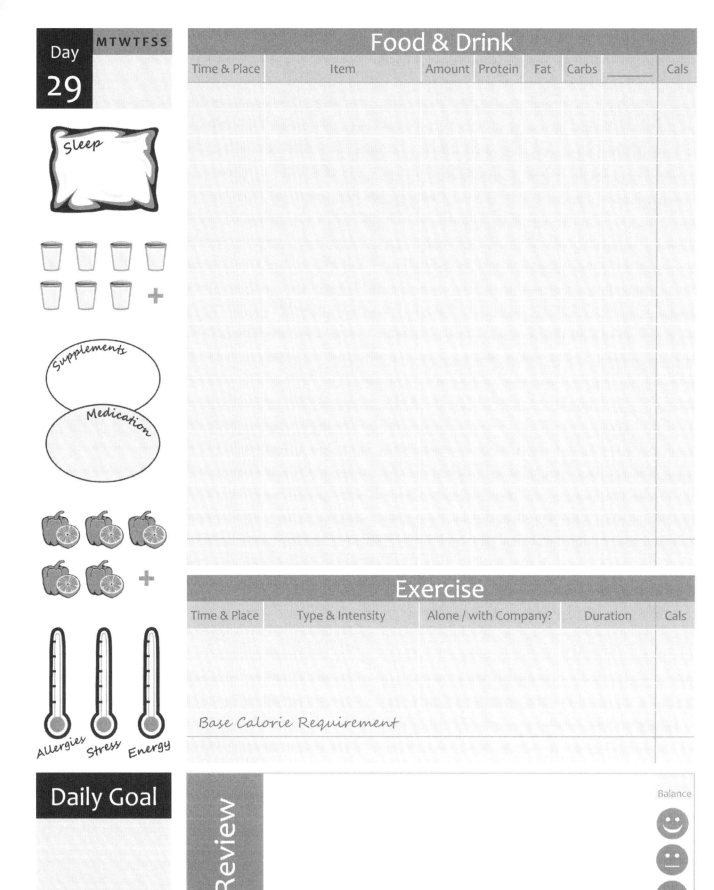

Day 29

MTWTFSS

Sleep

Supplements

Medication

Allergies Stress Energy

Daily Goal

X ✔

Food & Drink

Time & Place	Item	Amount	Protein	Fat	Carbs	_____	Cals

Exercise

Time & Place	Type & Intensity	Alone / with Company?	Duration	Cals

Base Calorie Requirement

Review

Balance

Food & Drink

Time & Place	Item	Amount	Protein	Fat	Carbs	_____	Cals

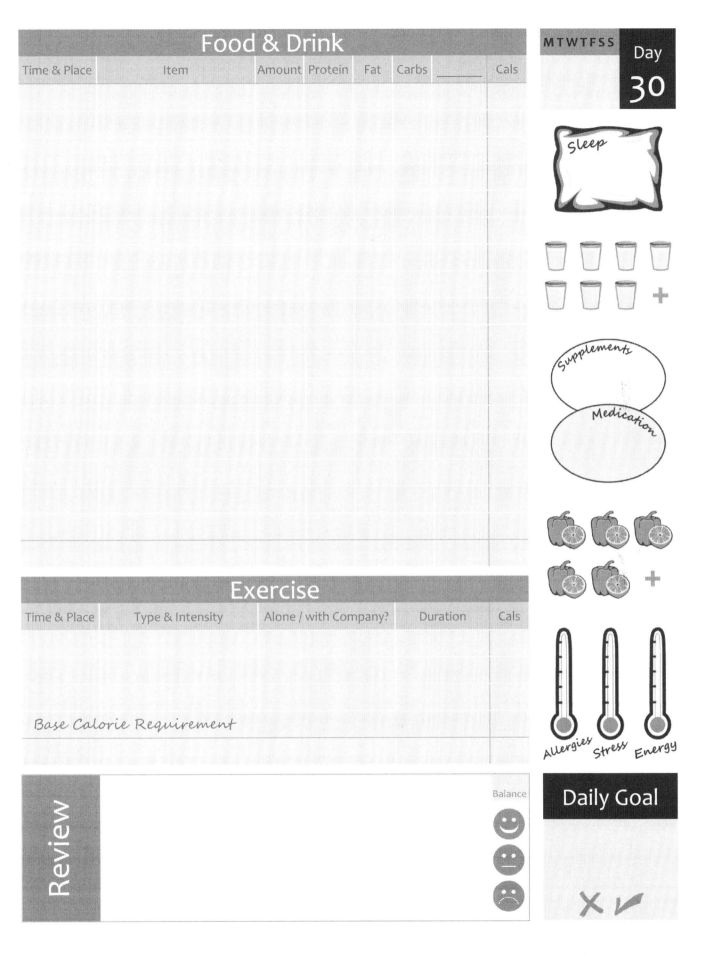

Sleep

Supplements

Medication

Exercise

Time & Place	Type & Intensity	Alone / with Company?	Duration	Cals
Base Calorie Requirement				

Allergies   Stress   Energy

Review

Balance

Daily Goal

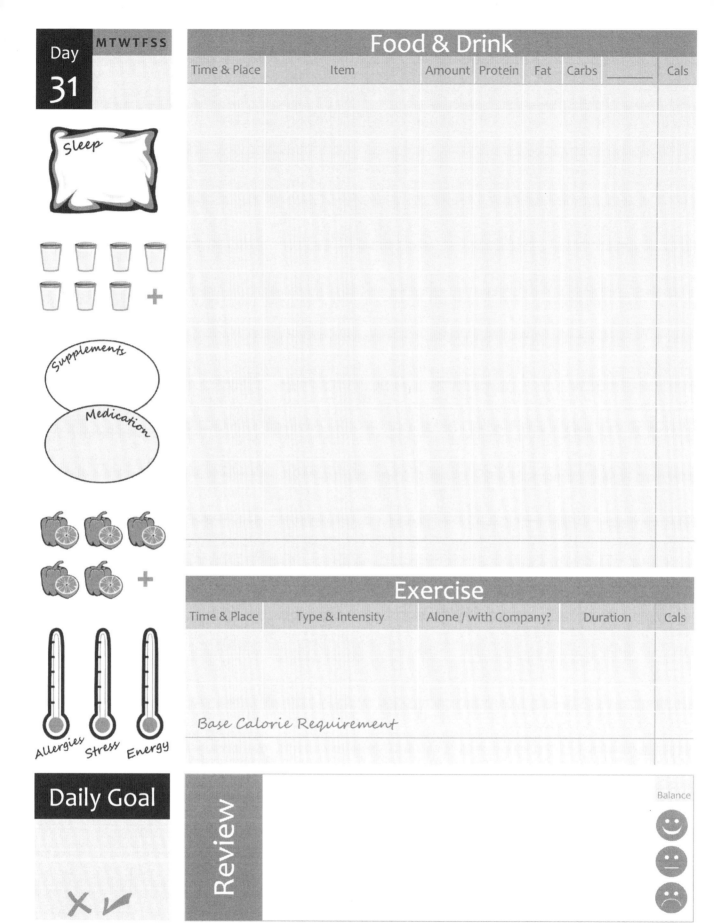

Day
31

MTWTFSS

Sleep

Supplements

Medication

Allergies Stress Energy

Daily Goal

X ✔

Food & Drink

Time & Place	Item	Amount	Protein	Fat	Carbs	_____	Cals

Exercise

Time & Place	Type & Intensity	Alone / with Company?	Duration	Cals
Base Calorie Requirement				

Review

Balance

Food & Drink

Time & Place	Item	Amount	Protein	Fat	Carbs	_____	Cals

Exercise

Time & Place	Type & Intensity	Alone / with Company?	Duration	Cals

Base Calorie Requirement

Review

Balance

Sleep

Supplements

Medication

Allergies   Stress   Energy

Daily Goal

X ✔

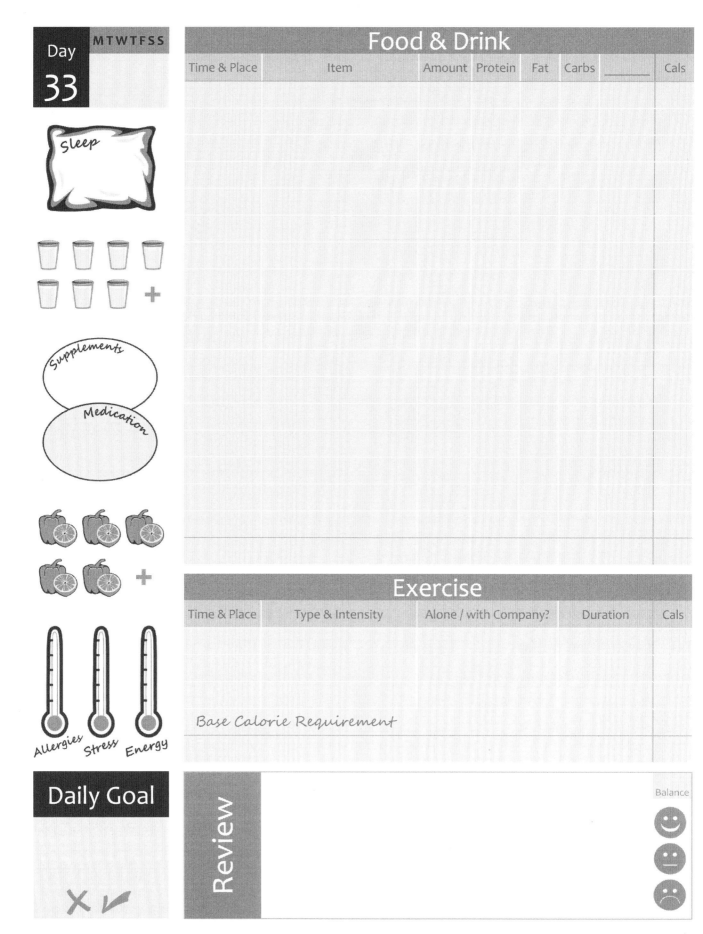

Day
33

MTWTFSS

Sleep

Supplements

Medication

Allergies Stress Energy

Daily Goal

X ✔

Food & Drink

Time & Place	Item	Amount	Protein	Fat	Carbs	_____	Cals

Exercise

Time & Place	Type & Intensity	Alone / with Company?	Duration	Cals
Base Calorie Requirement				

Review

Balance

Food & Drink

Time & Place	Item	Amount	Protein	Fat	Carbs	_____	Cals

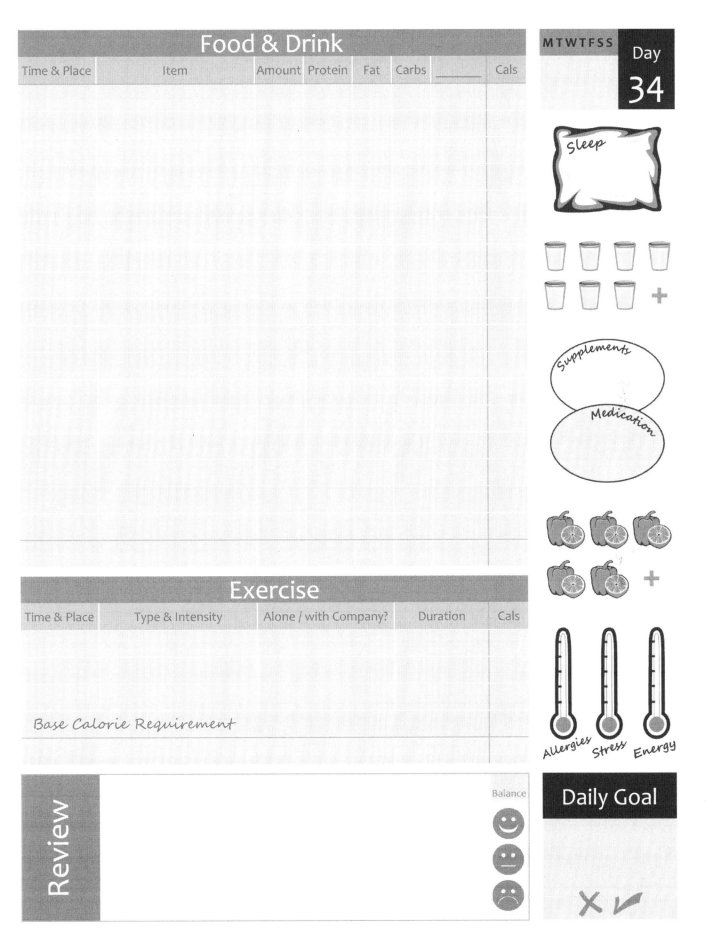

MTWTFSS

Day 34

Sleep

Supplements

Medication

Allergies Stress Energy

Exercise

Time & Place	Type & Intensity	Alone / with Company?	Duration	Cals

Base Calorie Requirement

Review

Balance

Daily Goal

X ✔

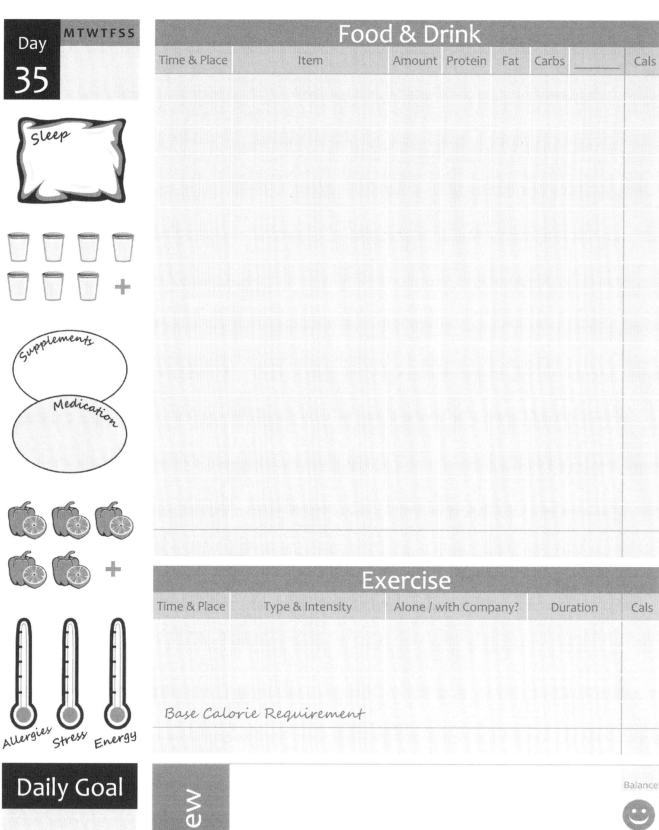

Day 35

MTWTFSS

Sleep

Supplements

Medication

Allergies   Stress   Energy

Daily Goal

X ✔

Food & Drink

Time & Place	Item	Amount	Protein	Fat	Carbs	_____	Cals

Exercise

Time & Place	Type & Intensity	Alone / with Company?	Duration	Cals
Base Calorie Requirement				

Review

Balance

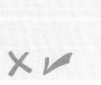

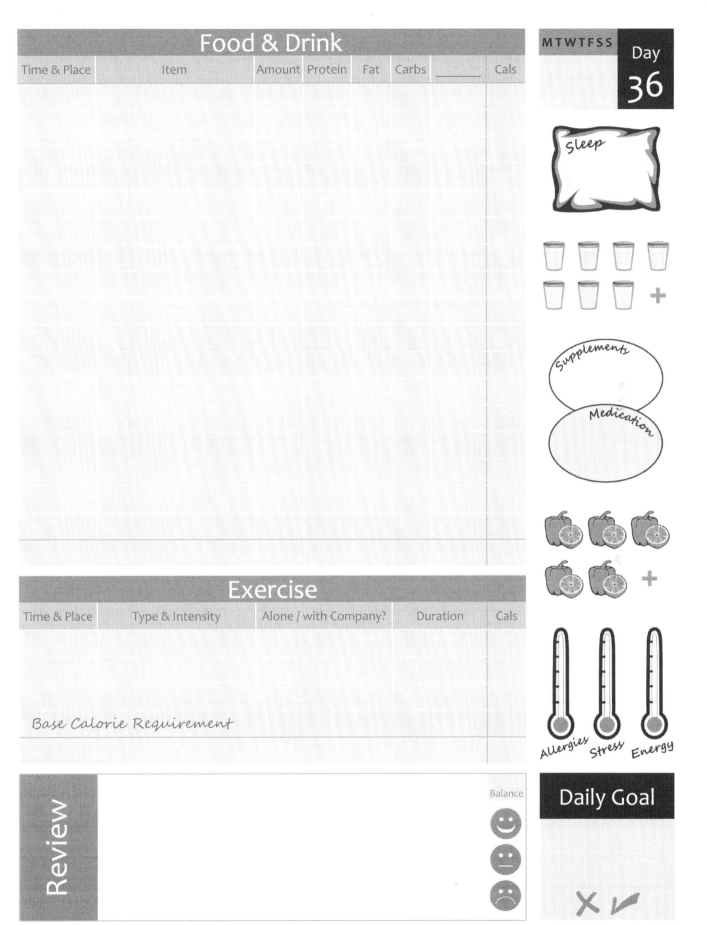

Food & Drink

Time & Place	Item	Amount	Protein	Fat	Carbs		Cals

Sleep

Supplements

Medication

Allergies Stress Energy

Exercise

Time & Place	Type & Intensity	Alone / with Company?	Duration	Cals
Base Calorie Requirement				

Review

Balance

Daily Goal

X ✔

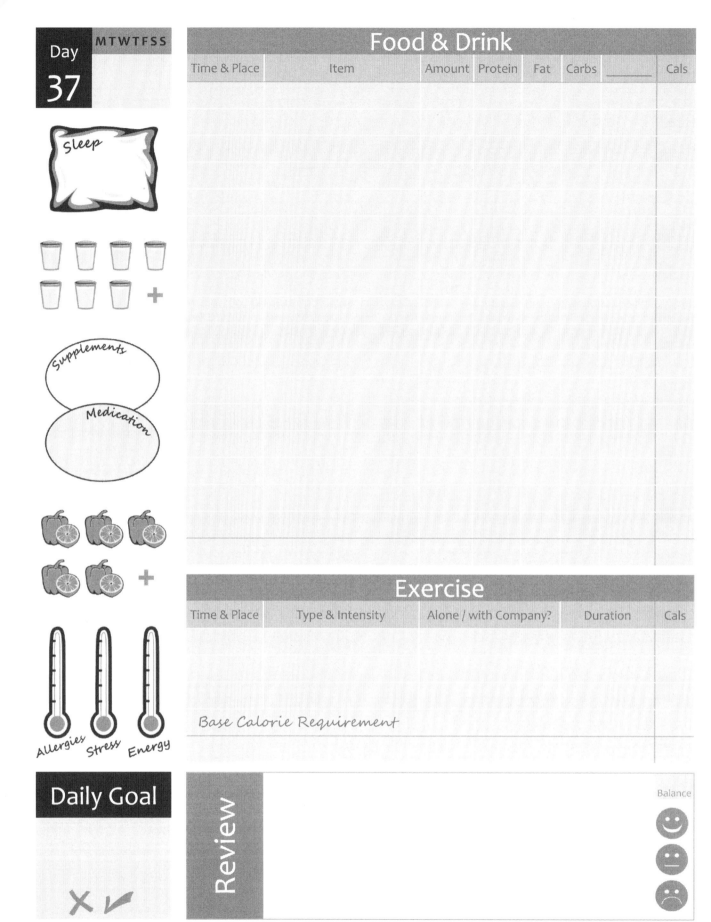

Day 37

MTWTFSS

Sleep

Supplements

Medication

Allergies Stress Energy

Daily Goal

X ✔

Food & Drink

Time & Place	Item	Amount	Protein	Fat	Carbs	_____	Cals

Exercise

Time & Place	Type & Intensity	Alone / with Company?	Duration	Cals

Base Calorie Requirement

Review

Balance

Food & Drink

Time & Place	Item	Amount	Protein	Fat	Carbs	_____	Cals

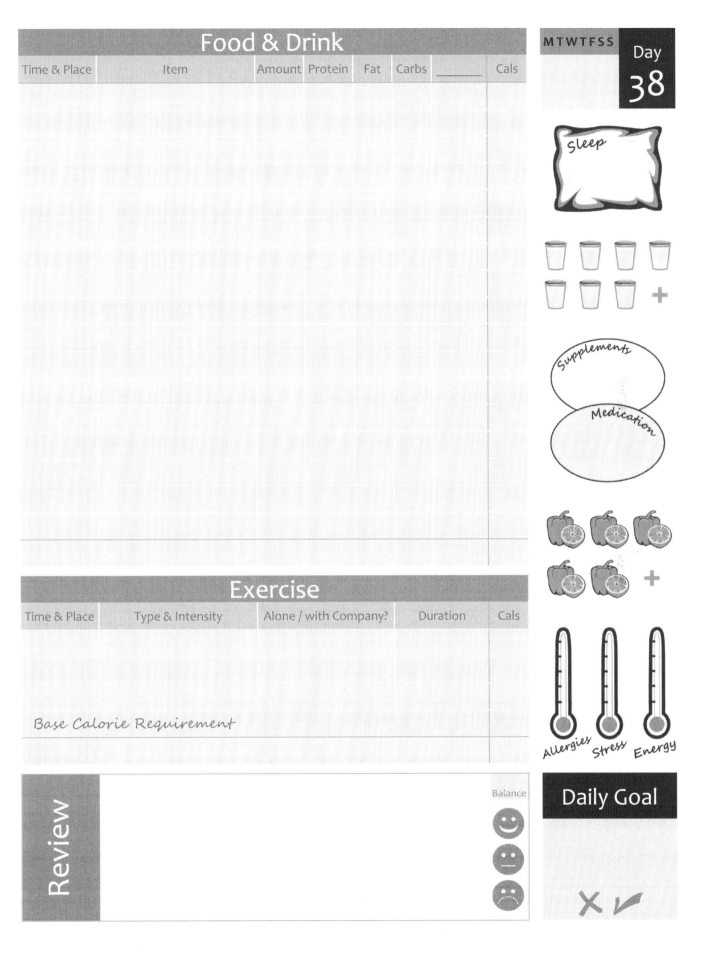

Sleep

Supplements

Medication

Allergies Stress Energy

Exercise

Time & Place	Type & Intensity	Alone / with Company?	Duration	Cals

Base Calorie Requirement

Review

Balance

Daily Goal

X ✔

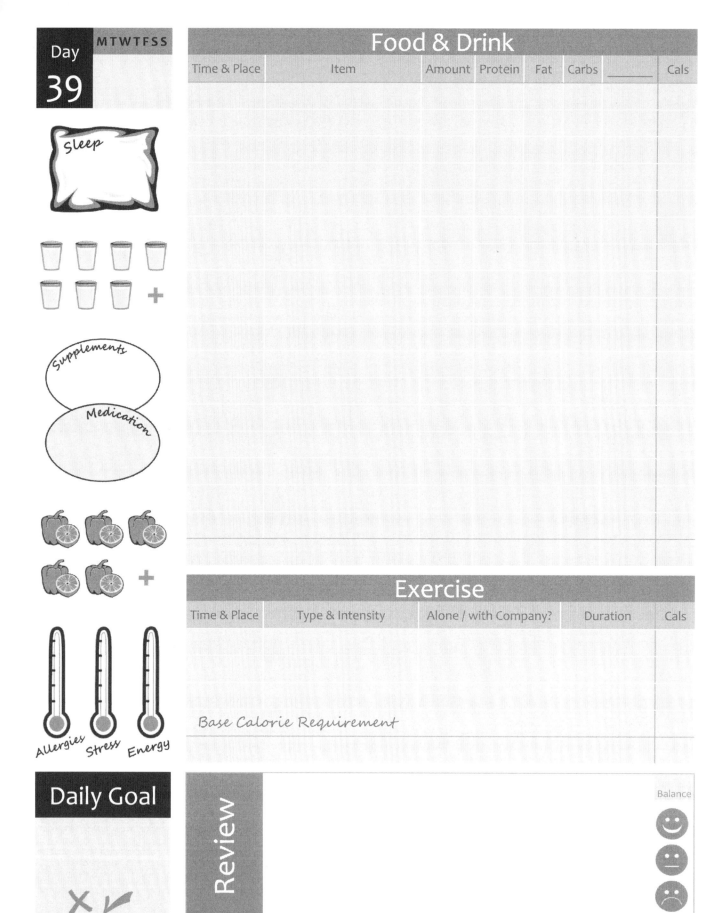

Day 39 MTWTFSS

Sleep

Supplements

Medication

Allergies Stress Energy

Daily Goal

X ✔

Food & Drink

Time & Place	Item	Amount	Protein	Fat	Carbs	_____	Cals

Exercise

Time & Place	Type & Intensity	Alone / with Company?	Duration	Cals

Base Calorie Requirement

Review

Balance

😊

😐

☹️

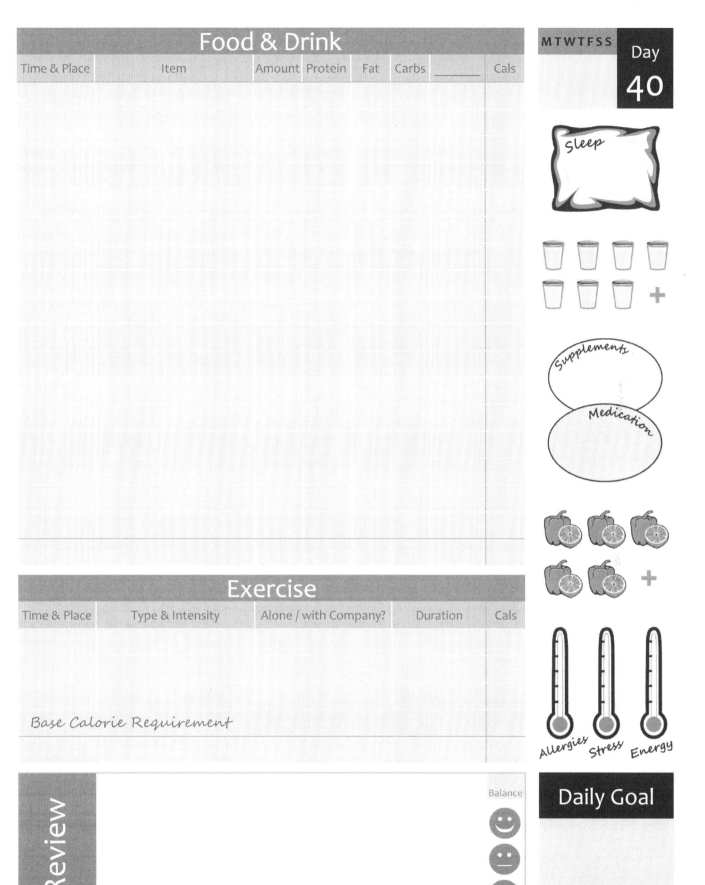

Food & Drink

Time & Place	Item	Amount	Protein	Fat	Carbs	____	Cals

Exercise

Time & Place	Type & Intensity	Alone / with Company?	Duration	Cals

Base Calorie Requirement

Review

Balance

MTWTFSS

Day

40

Sleep

Supplements

Medication

Allergies   Stress   Energy

Daily Goal

X ✔

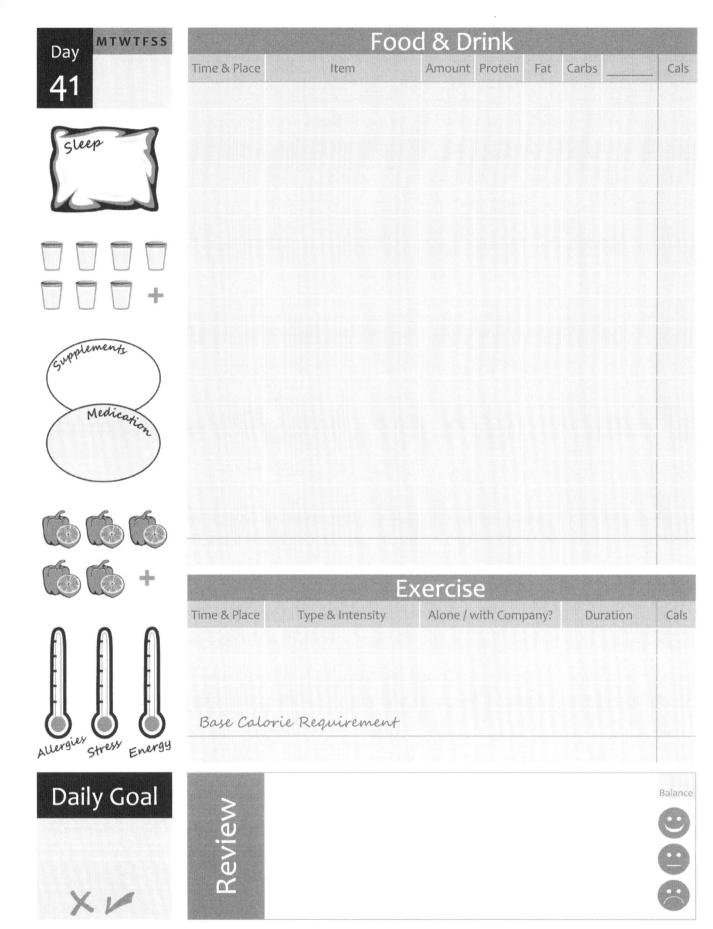

Day 41

MTWTFSS

Sleep

Supplements

Medication

Allergies Stress Energy

Daily Goal

X ✔

Food & Drink

Time & Place	Item	Amount	Protein	Fat	Carbs	_____	Cals

Exercise

Time & Place	Type & Intensity	Alone / with Company?	Duration	Cals

Base Calorie Requirement

Review

Balance

Food & Drink

Time & Place	Item	Amount	Protein	Fat	Carbs	_____	Cals

Exercise

Time & Place	Type & Intensity	Alone / with Company?	Duration	Cals

Base Calorie Requirement

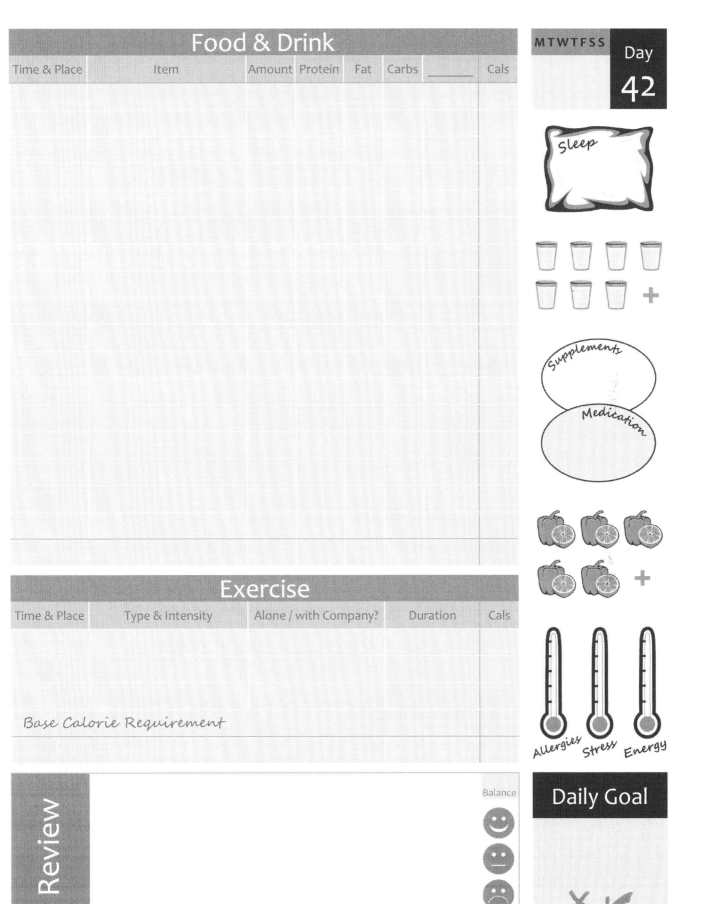

Sleep

Supplements

Medication

Allergies   Stress   Energy

Review

Balance

Daily Goal

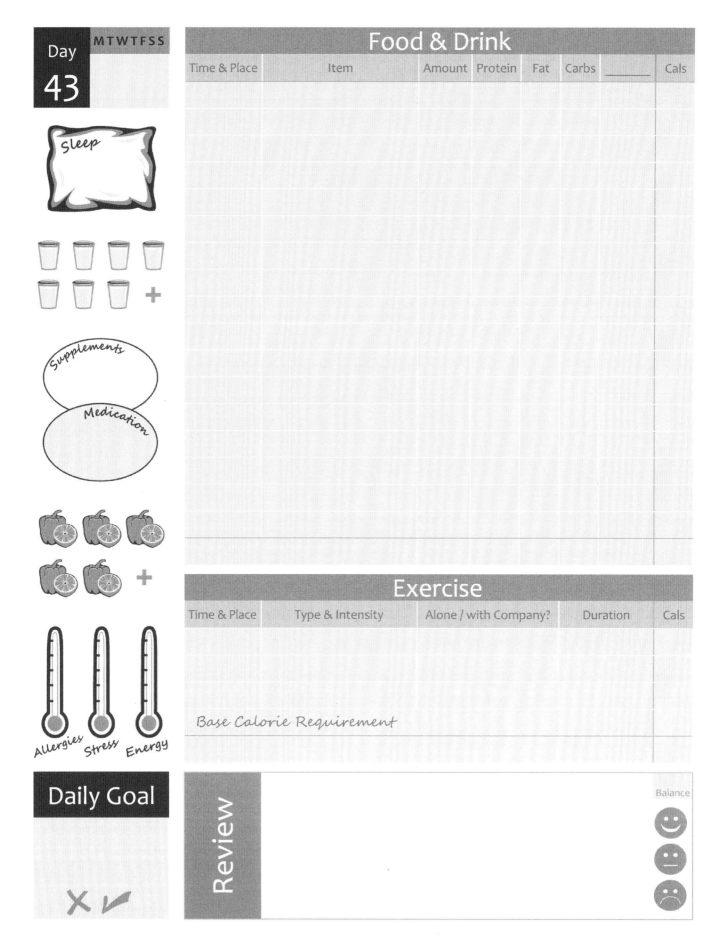

Sleep

Supplements

Medication

Allergies   Stress   Energy

Daily Goal

X ✔

Food & Drink

Time & Place	Item	Amount	Protein	Fat	Carbs		Cals

Exercise

Time & Place	Type & Intensity	Alone / with Company?	Duration	Cals
Base Calorie Requirement				

Review

Balance

Food & Drink

Time & Place	Item	Amount	Protein	Fat	Carbs	_____	Cals

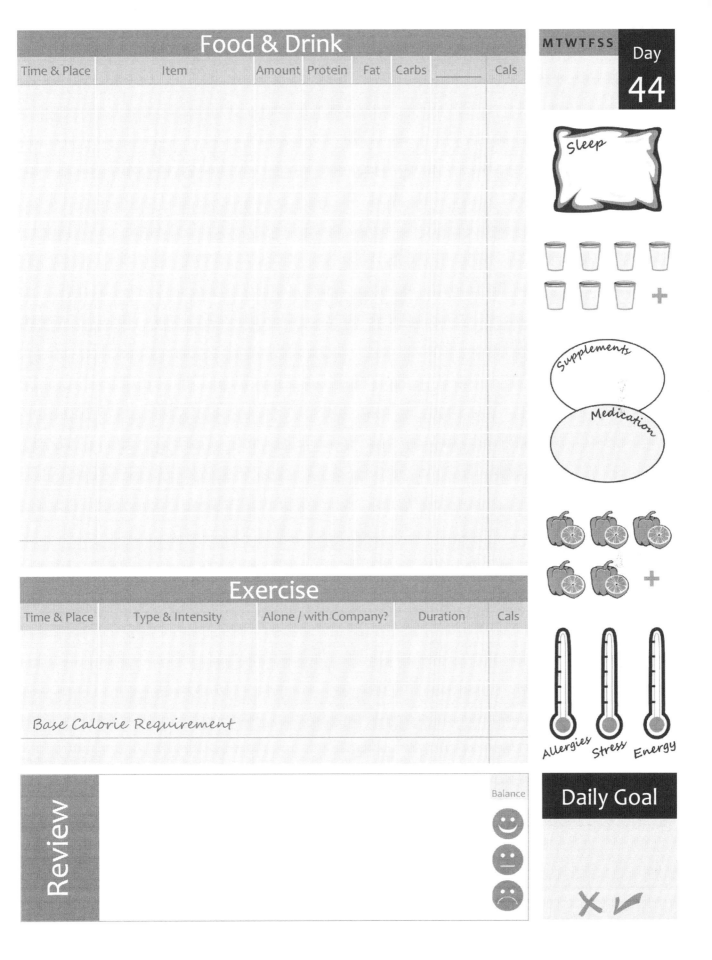

Sleep

Supplements

Medication

Exercise

Time & Place	Type & Intensity	Alone / with Company?	Duration	Cals
Base Calorie Requirement				

Allergies Stress Energy

Review

Balance

Daily Goal

✗ ✔

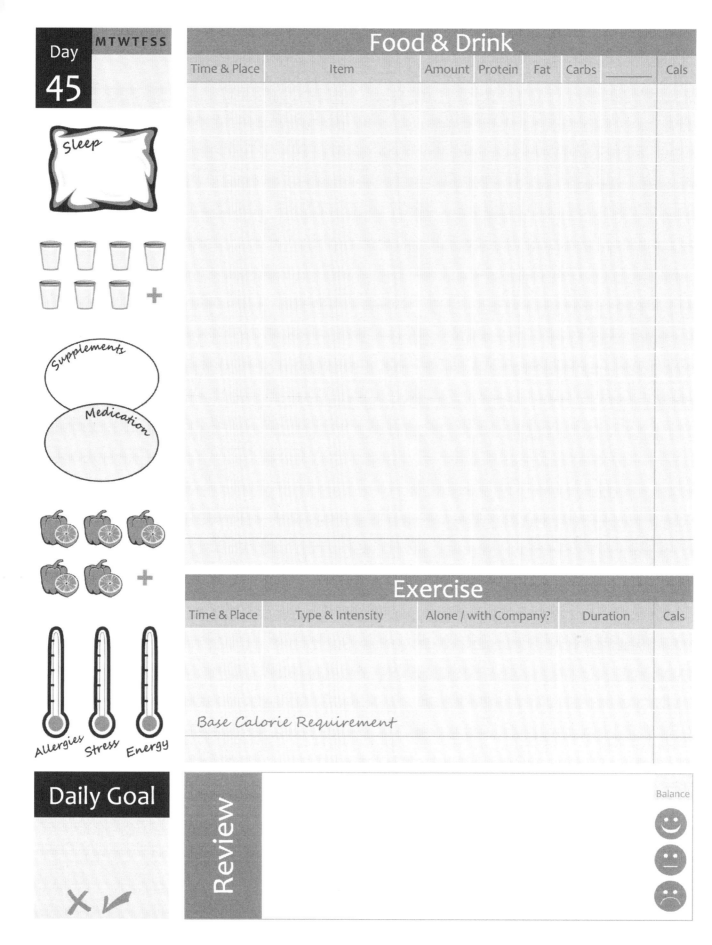

Day 45

MTWTFSS

Sleep

Supplements

Medication

Allergies Stress Energy

Daily Goal

✗ ✔

Food & Drink

Time & Place	Item	Amount	Protein	Fat	Carbs	_____	Cals

Exercise

Time & Place	Type & Intensity	Alone / with Company?	Duration	Cals
Base Calorie Requirement				

Review

Balance

🙂
😐
🙁

Food & Drink

Time & Place	Item	Amount	Protein	Fat	Carbs		Cals

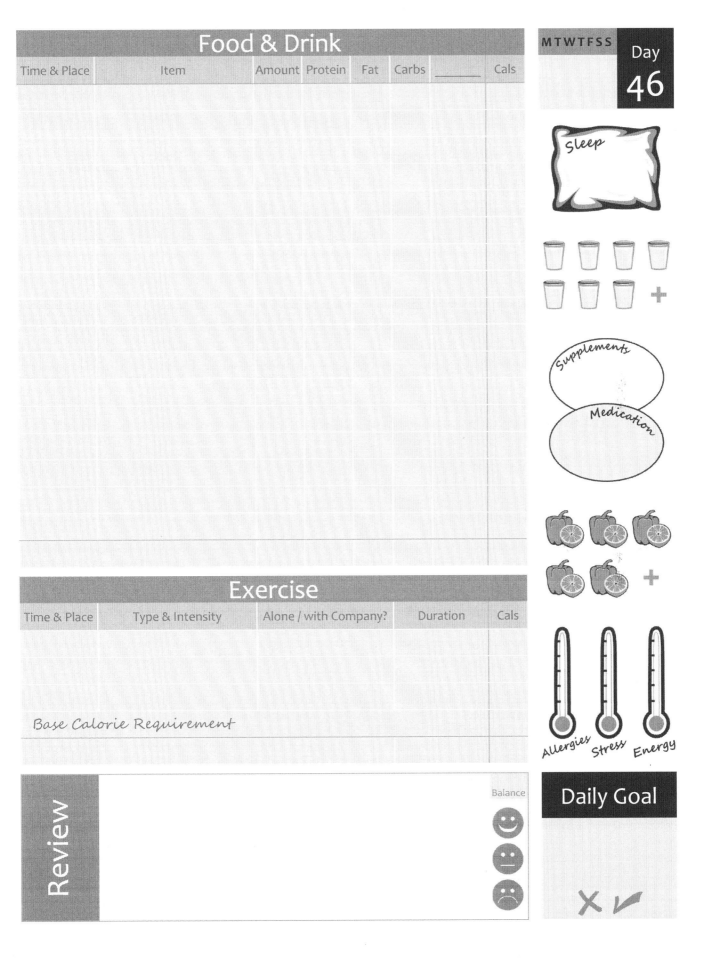

Sleep

Supplements

Medication

Exercise

Time & Place	Type & Intensity	Alone / with Company?	Duration	Cals

Base Calorie Requirement

Allergies   Stress   Energy

Review

Balance

Daily Goal

X ✔

Day 47

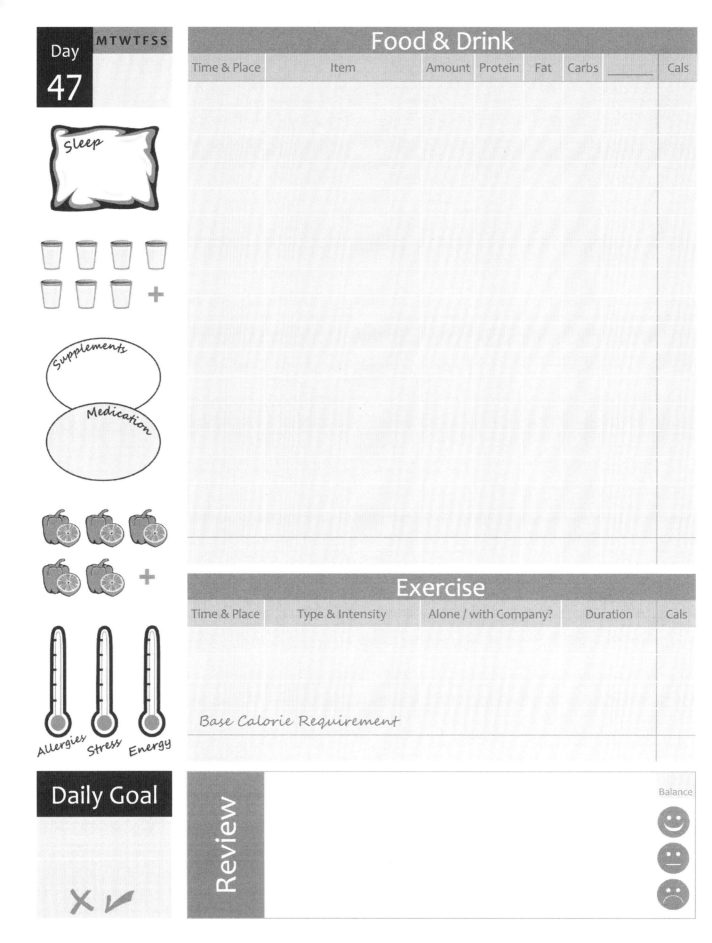

Sleep

Supplements

Medication

Allergies   Stress   Energy

Daily Goal

X ✔

Food & Drink

Time & Place	Item	Amount	Protein	Fat	Carbs	_____	Cals

Exercise

Time & Place	Type & Intensity	Alone / with Company?	Duration	Cals
Base Calorie Requirement				

Review

Balance

☺
😐
☹

Food & Drink

Time & Place	Item	Amount	Protein	Fat	Carbs	_____	Cals

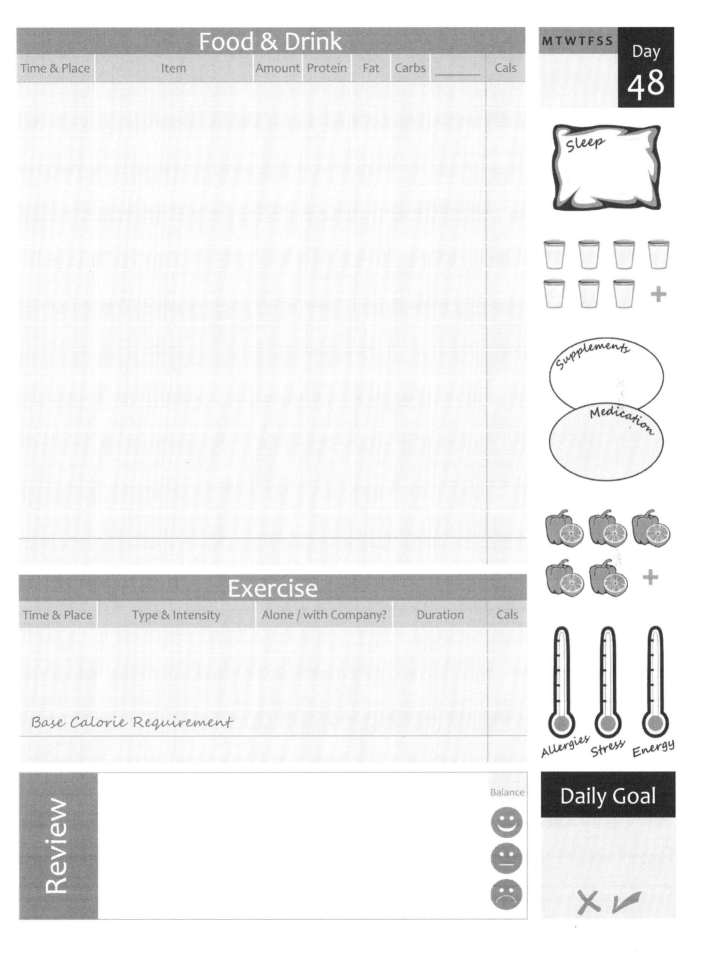

Sleep

Supplements

Medication

Exercise

Time & Place	Type & Intensity	Alone / with Company?	Duration	Cals
Base Calorie Requirement				

Allergies Stress Energy

Review

Balance

Daily Goal

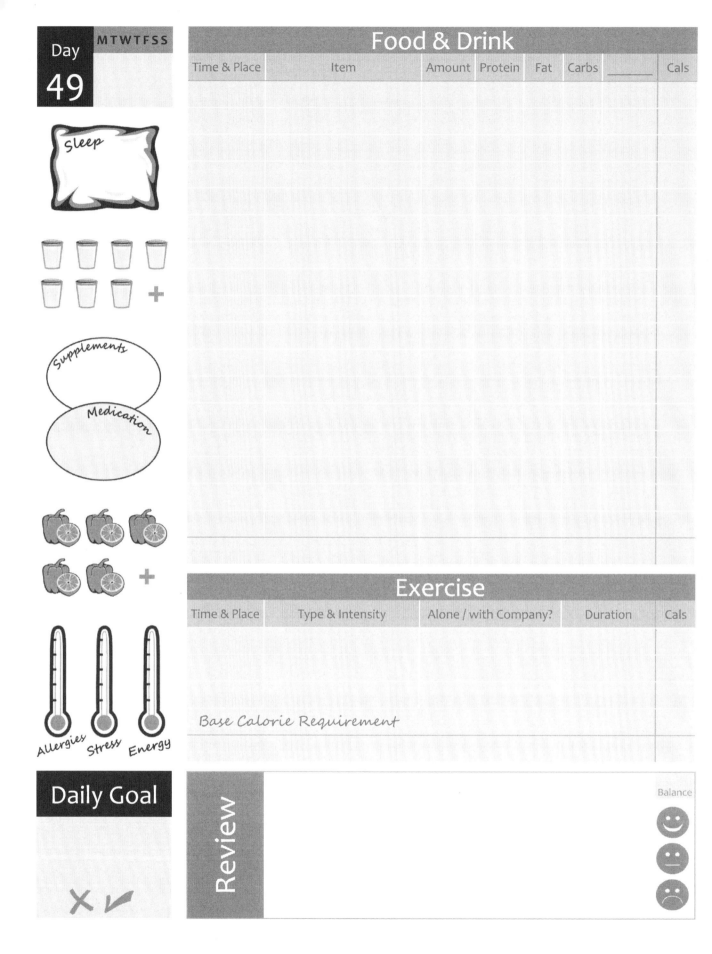

Day 49

MTWTFSS

Sleep

Supplements

Medication

Allergies Stress Energy

Daily Goal

X ✔

Food & Drink

Time & Place	Item	Amount	Protein	Fat	Carbs	_____	Cals

Exercise

Time & Place	Type & Intensity	Alone / with Company?	Duration	Cals

Base Calorie Requirement

Review

Balance

Food & Drink

Time & Place	Item	Amount	Protein	Fat	Carbs	___	Cals

Sleep

Supplements

Medication

Exercise

Time & Place	Type & Intensity	Alone / with Company?	Duration	Cals
Base Calorie Requirement				

Allergies Stress Energy

Review

Balance

Daily Goal

X ✓

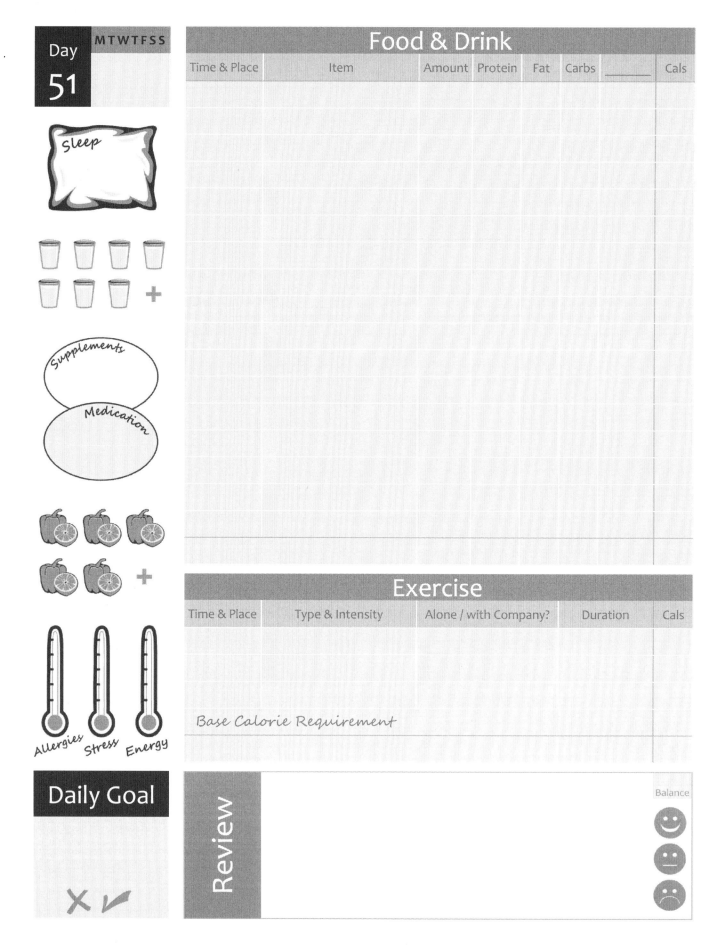

Day 51

MTWTFSS

Sleep

Supplements

Medication

Allergies Stress Energy

Daily Goal

X ✔

Food & Drink

Time & Place	Item	Amount	Protein	Fat	Carbs	_____	Cals

Exercise

Time & Place	Type & Intensity	Alone / with Company?	Duration	Cals

Base Calorie Requirement

Review

Balance

Food & Drink

Time & Place	Item	Amount	Protein	Fat	Carbs	_____	Cals

Sleep

Supplements

Medication

Exercise

Time & Place	Type & Intensity	Alone / with Company?	Duration	Cals
Base Calorie Requirement				

Allergies   Stress   Energy

Review

Balance

Daily Goal

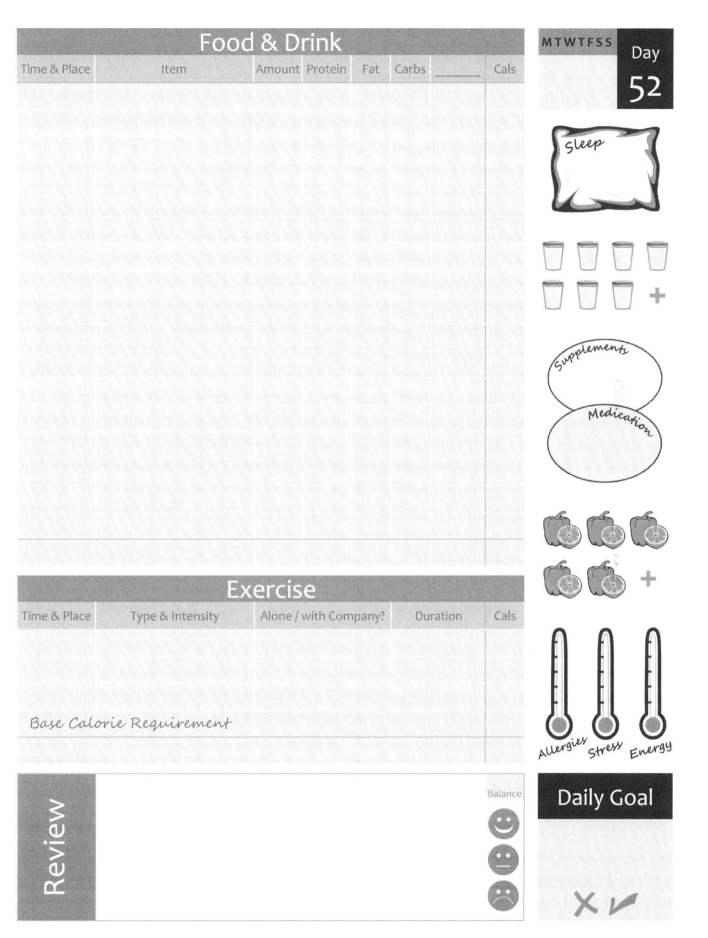

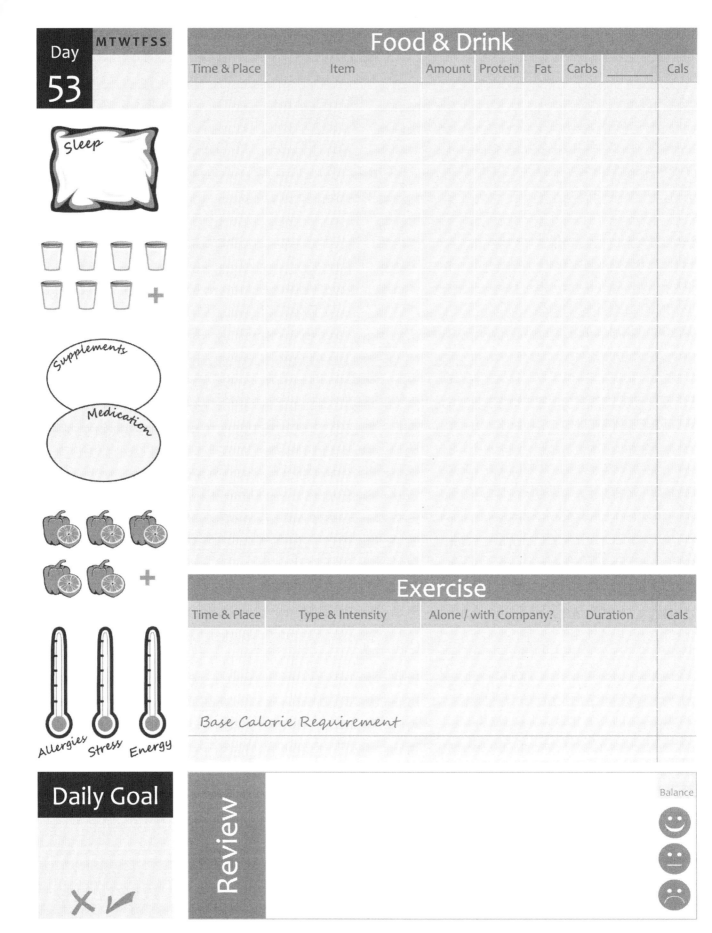

Day
53

MTWTFSS

Sleep

Supplements

Medication

Allergies   Stress   Energy

Daily Goal

X ✔

Food & Drink

Time & Place	Item	Amount	Protein	Fat	Carbs	_____	Cals

Exercise

Time & Place	Type & Intensity	Alone / with Company?	Duration	Cals
Base Calorie Requirement				

Review

Balance

Food & Drink

Time & Place	Item	Amount	Protein	Fat	Carbs	_____	Cals

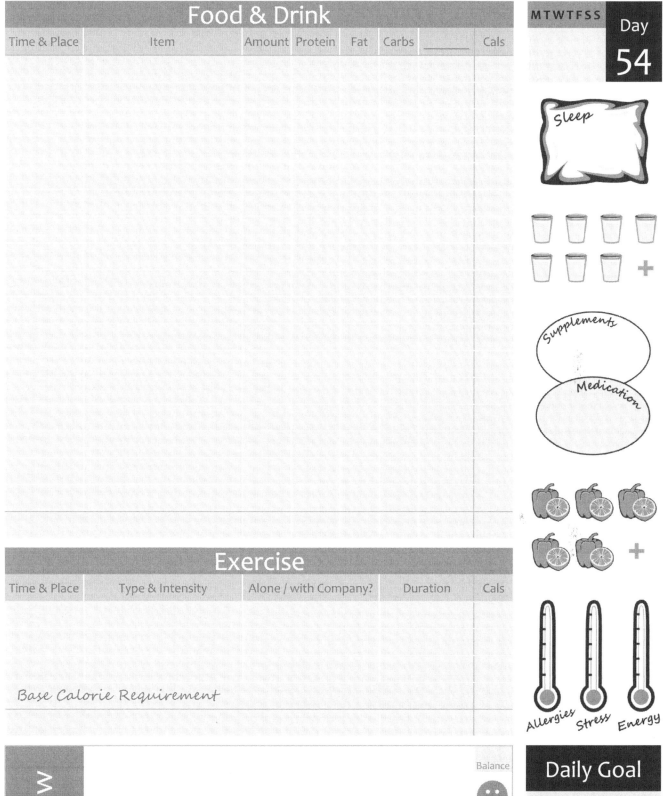

Sleep

Supplements

Medication

Exercise

Time & Place	Type & Intensity	Alone / with Company?	Duration	Cals
Base Calorie Requirement				

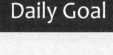

Allergies   Stress   Energy

Review

Balance

Daily Goal

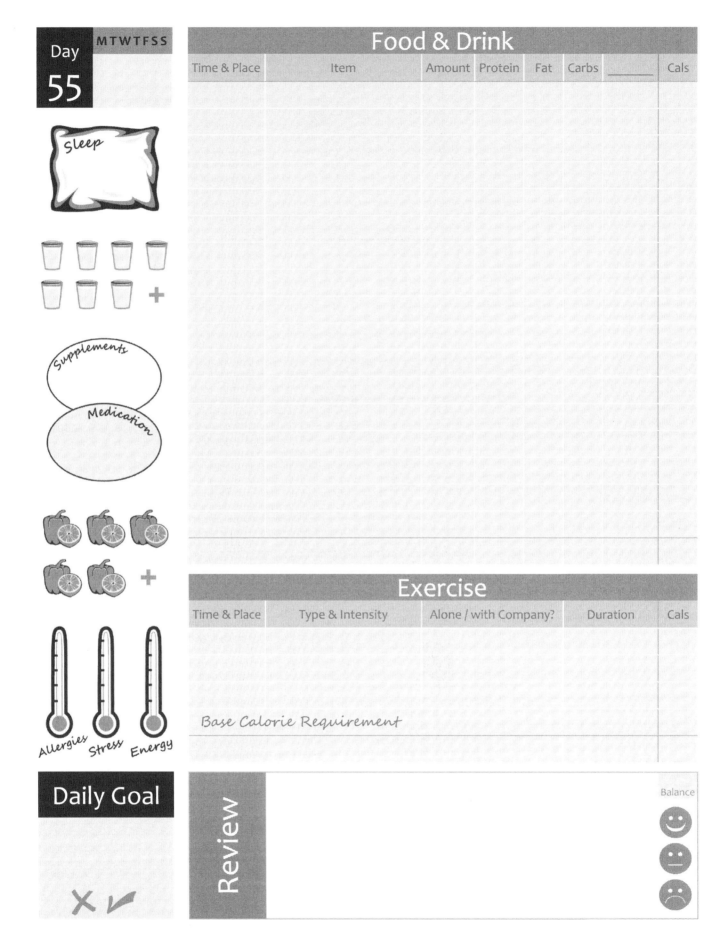

Day 55

M T W T F S S

Sleep

Supplements

Medication

Allergies Stress Energy

Daily Goal

X ✔

Food & Drink

Time & Place	Item	Amount	Protein	Fat	Carbs		Cals

Exercise

Time & Place	Type & Intensity	Alone / with Company?	Duration	Cals
Base Calorie Requirement				

Review

Balance

Food & Drink

Time & Place	Item	Amount	Protein	Fat	Carbs	_____	Cals

Sleep

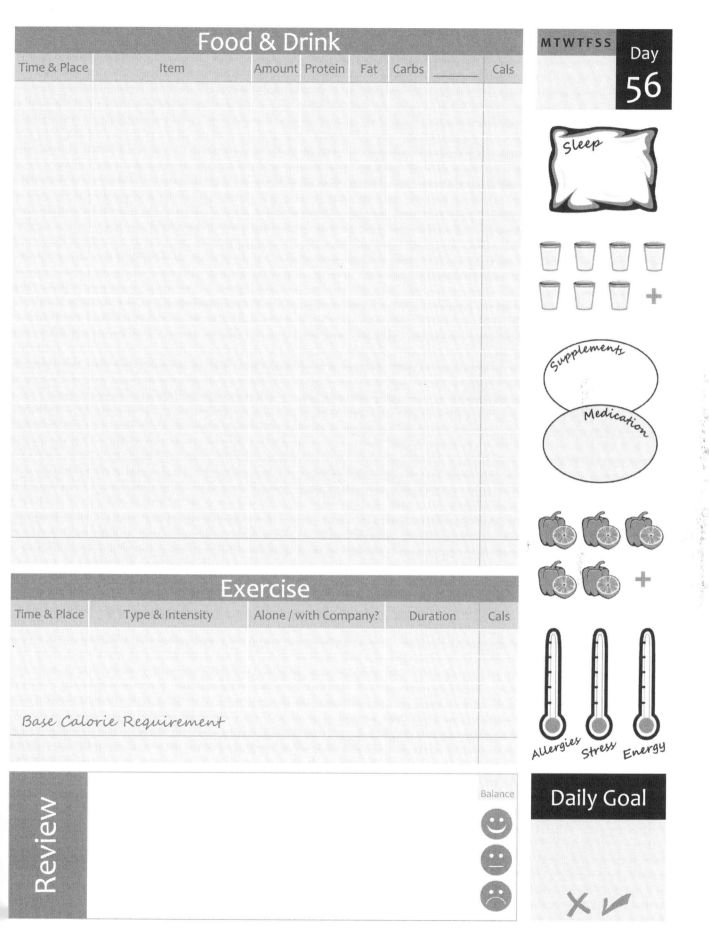

Supplements

Medication

Exercise

Time & Place	Type & Intensity	Alone / with Company?	Duration	Cals

Base Calorie Requirement

Allergies   Stress   Energy

Review

Balance

Daily Goal

X ✔

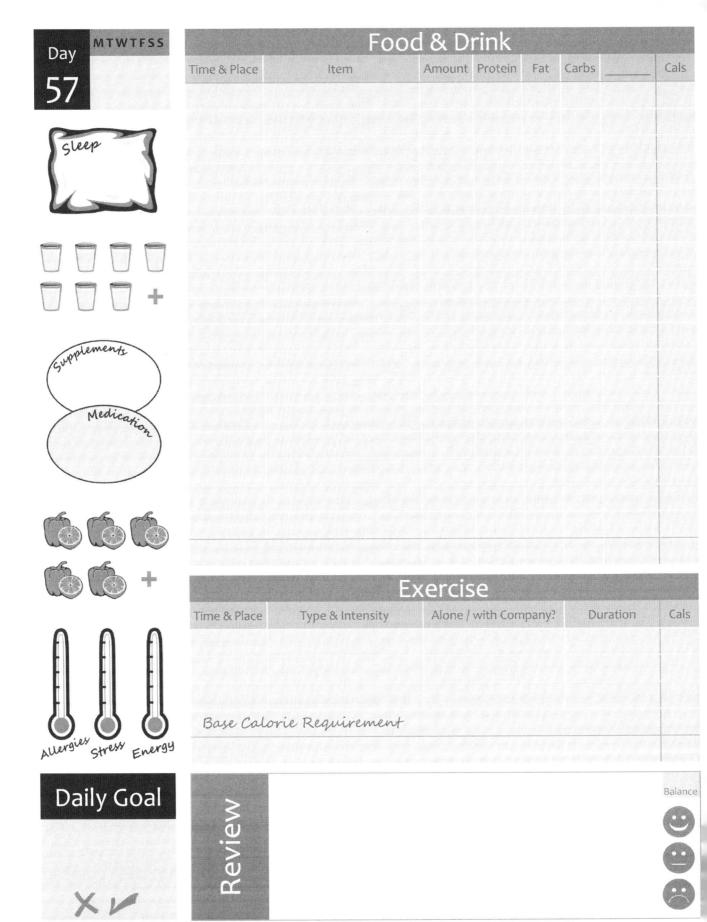

Day
57

MTWTFSS

Sleep

Supplements

Medication

Allergies Stress Energy

Daily Goal

X ✔

Food & Drink

Time & Place	Item	Amount	Protein	Fat	Carbs	_____	Cals

Exercise

Time & Place	Type & Intensity	Alone / with Company?	Duration	Cals
Base Calorie Requirement				

Review

Balance

Food & Drink

Time & Place	Item	Amount	Protein	Fat	Carbs	_____	Cals

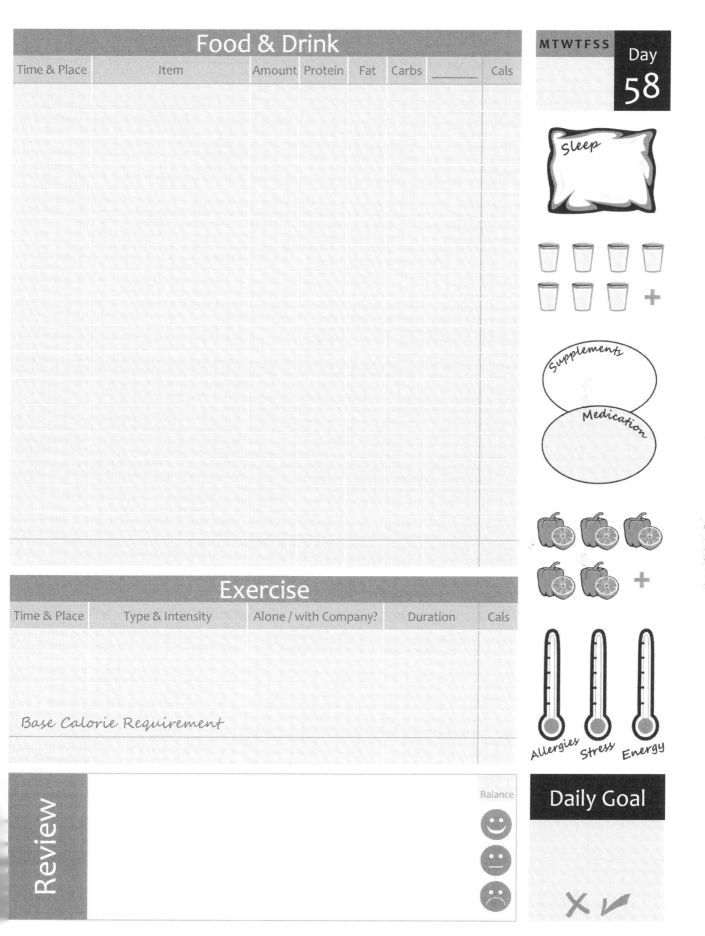

Sleep

Supplements

Medication

Exercise

Time & Place	Type & Intensity	Alone / with Company?	Duration	Cals
Base Calorie Requirement				

Allergies Stress Energy

Review

Balance

Daily Goal

X ✔

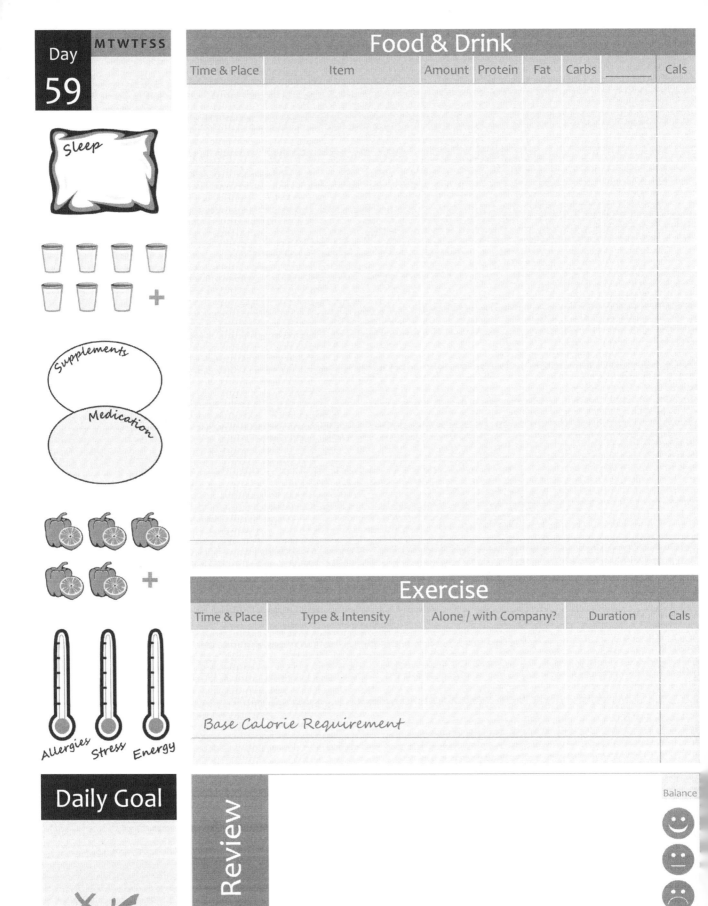

Day
59

MTWTFSS

Sleep

Supplements

Medication

Allergies Stress Energy

Daily Goal

X ✔

Food & Drink

Time & Place	Item	Amount	Protein	Fat	Carbs	_____	Cals

Exercise

Time & Place	Type & Intensity	Alone / with Company?	Duration	Cals
Base Calorie Requirement				

Review

Balance

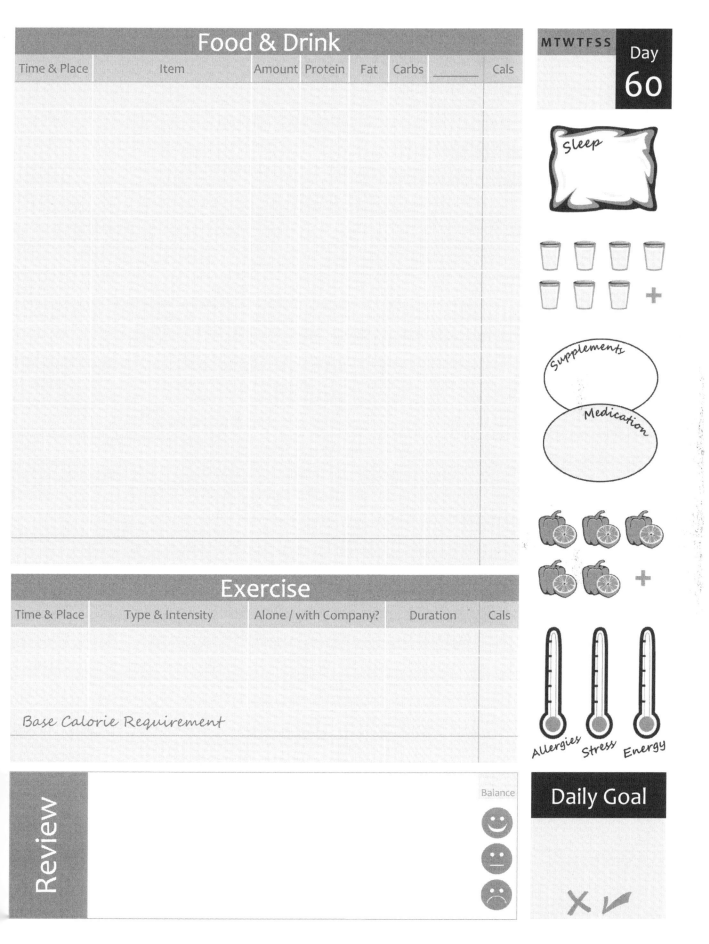

Food & Drink

Time & Place	Item	Amount	Protein	Fat	Carbs	_____	Cals

Sleep

Supplements

Medication

Allergies   Stress   Energy

Exercise

Time & Place	Type & Intensity	Alone / with Company?	Duration	Cals
Base Calorie Requirement				

Review

Balance

Daily Goal

X ✔

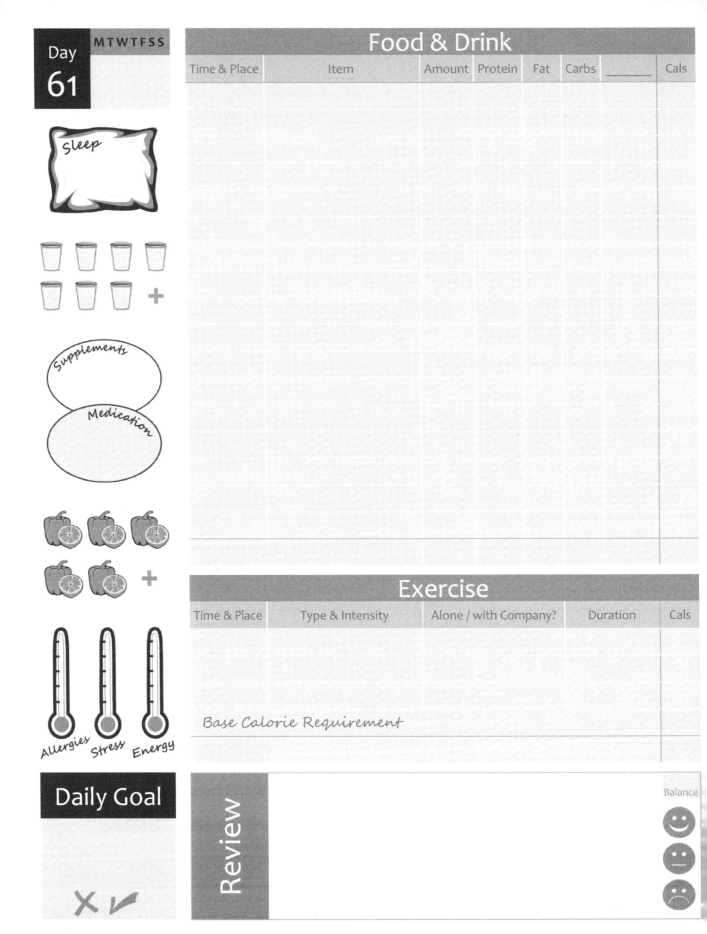

Day 61

MTWTFSS

Sleep

Supplements

Medication

Allergies Stress Energy

Daily Goal

X ✔

Food & Drink

Time & Place	Item	Amount	Protein	Fat	Carbs		Cals

Exercise

Time & Place	Type & Intensity	Alone / with Company?	Duration	Cals
Base Calorie Requirement				

Review

Balance

Food & Drink

Time & Place	Item	Amount	Protein	Fat	Carbs	_____	Cals

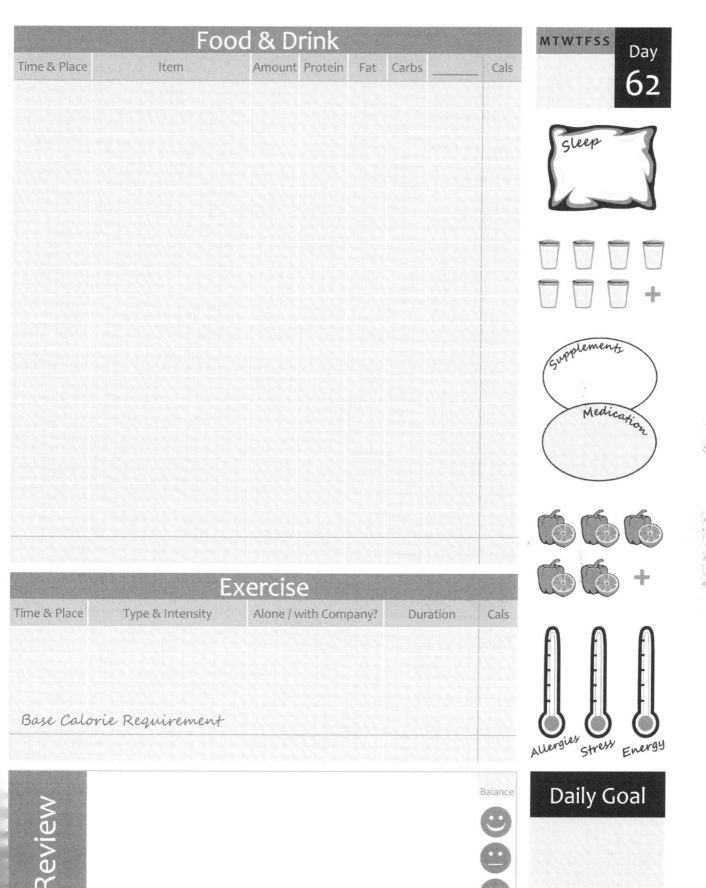

MTWTFSS

Day
62

Sleep

Supplements

Medication

Allergies   Stress   Energy

Exercise

Time & Place	Type & Intensity	Alone / with Company?	Duration	Cals
Base Calorie Requirement				

Review

Balance

Daily Goal

✗ ✓

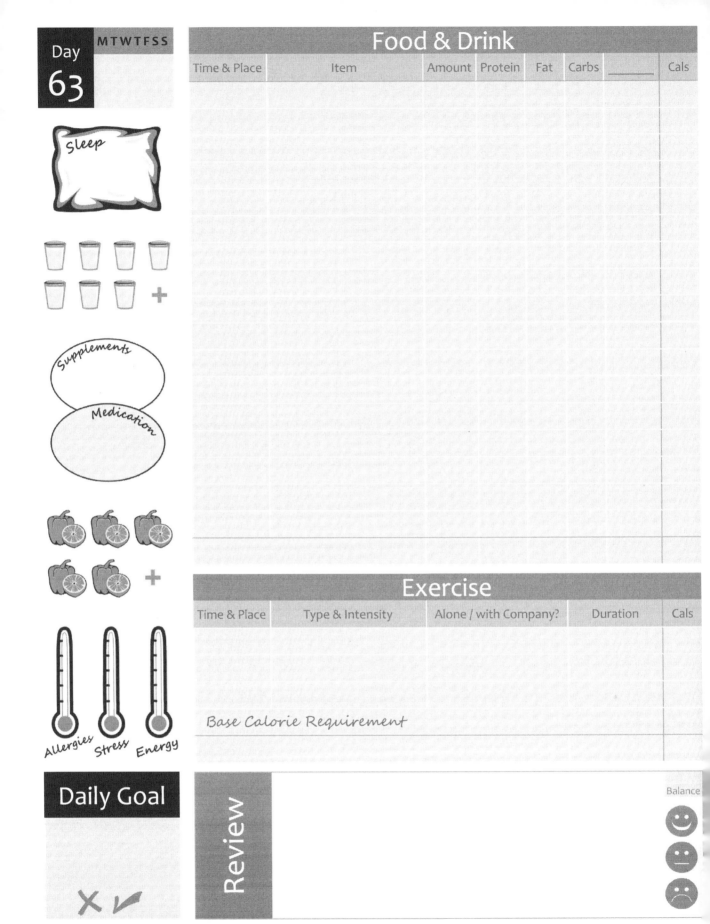

Food & Drink

Time & Place	Item	Amount	Protein	Fat	Carbs	_____	Cals

Exercise

Time & Place	Type & Intensity	Alone / with Company?	Duration	Cals

Base Calorie Requirement

Day
63

MTWTFSS

Sleep

Supplements

Medication

Allergies   Stress   Energy

Daily Goal

X ✔

Review

Balance

🙂

😐

☹️

Food & Drink

Time & Place	Item	Amount	Protein	Fat	Carbs	_____	Cals

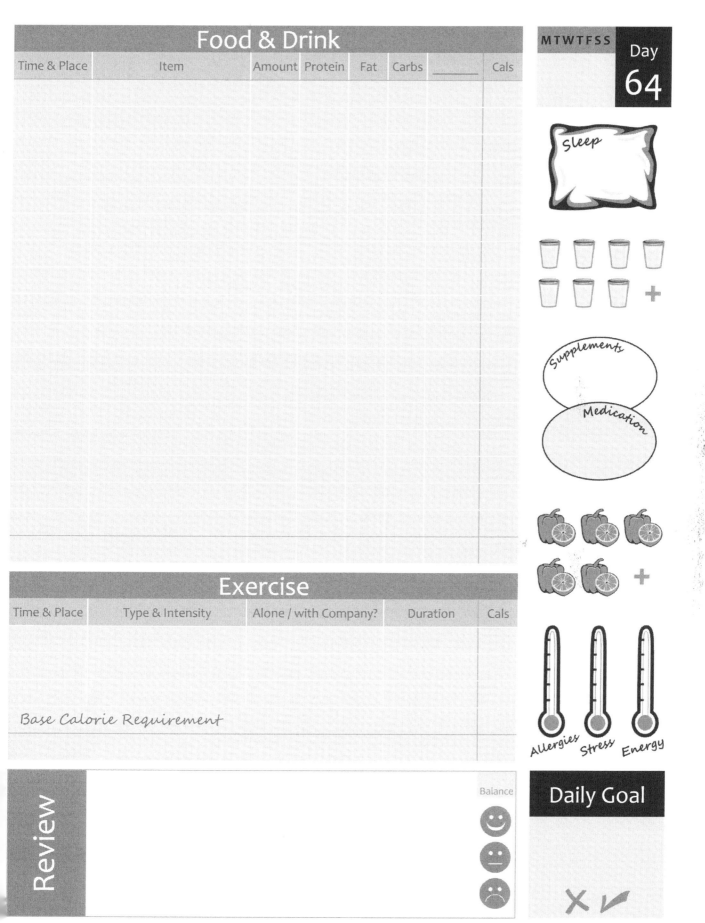

Sleep

Supplements

Medication

Exercise

Time & Place	Type & Intensity	Alone / with Company?	Duration	Cals
Base Calorie Requirement				

Allergies   Stress   Energy

Review

Balance

Daily Goal

Sleep

Supplements

Medication

Allergies Stress Energy

Daily Goal

Food & Drink

Time & Place	Item	Amount	Protein	Fat	Carbs	_____	Cals

Exercise

Time & Place	Type & Intensity	Alone / with Company?	Duration	Cals
Base Calorie Requirement				

Review

Balance

Food & Drink

Time & Place	Item	Amount	Protein	Fat	Carbs	_____	Cals

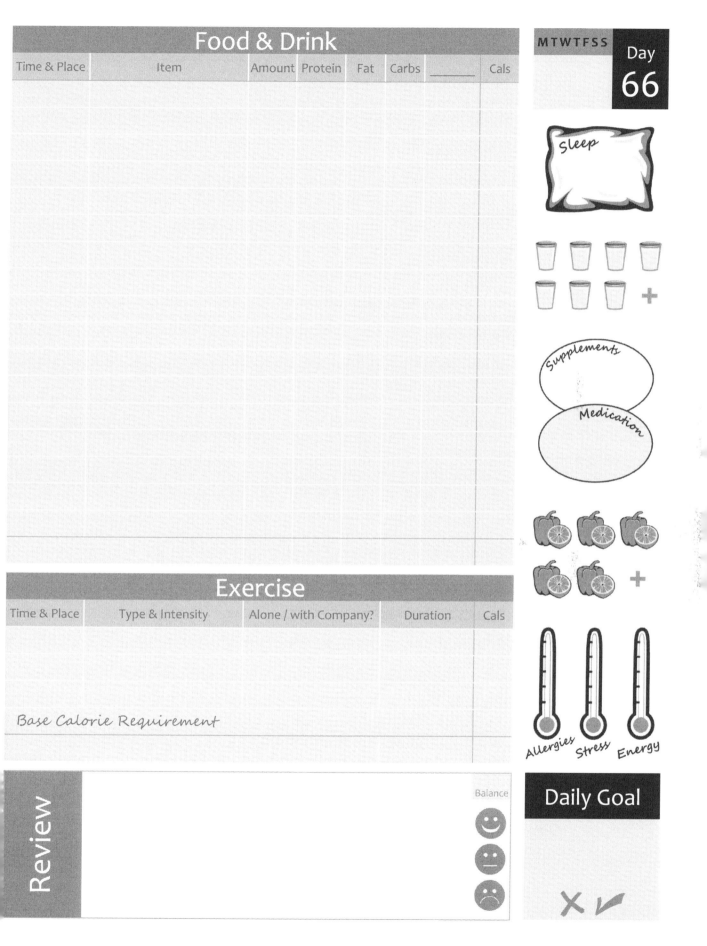

Sleep

Supplements

Medication

Exercise

Time & Place	Type & Intensity	Alone / with Company?	Duration	Cals

Base Calorie Requirement

Allergies Stress Energy

Review

Balance

Daily Goal

X ✔

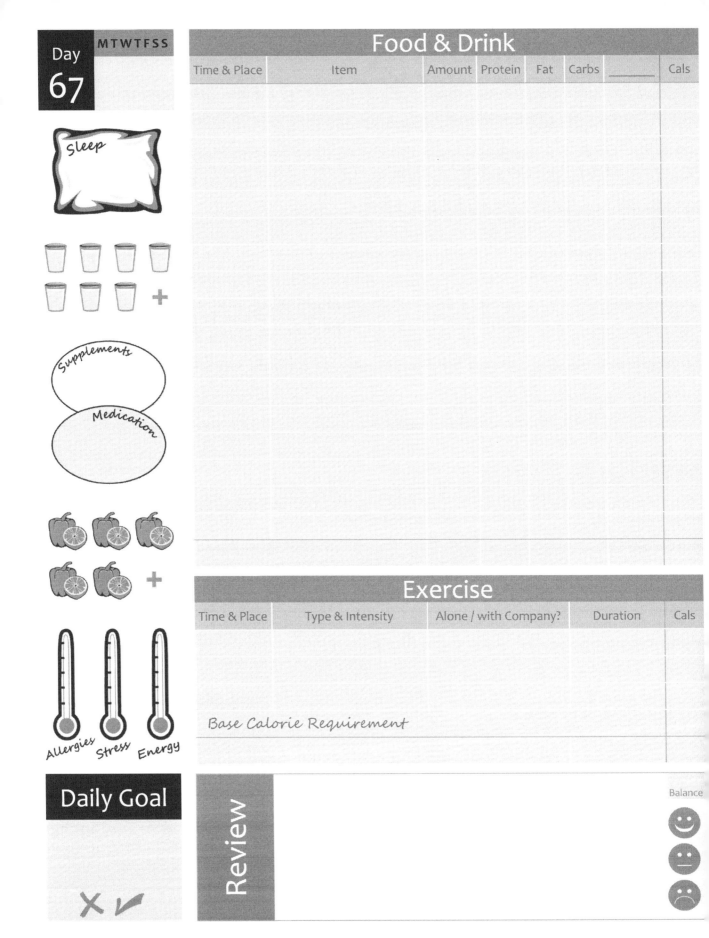

Day
67

MTWTFSS

Sleep

Supplements

Medication

Allergies Stress Energy

Daily Goal

X ✓

Food & Drink

Time & Place	Item	Amount	Protein	Fat	Carbs	_____	Cals

Exercise

Time & Place	Type & Intensity	Alone / with Company?	Duration	Cals

Base Calorie Requirement

Review

Balance

Food & Drink

Time & Place	Item	Amount	Protein	Fat	Carbs	_____	Cals

Sleep

Supplements

Medication

Exercise

Time & Place	Type & Intensity	Alone / with Company?	Duration	Cals

Base Calorie Requirement

Allergies Stress Energy

Review

Balance

Daily Goal

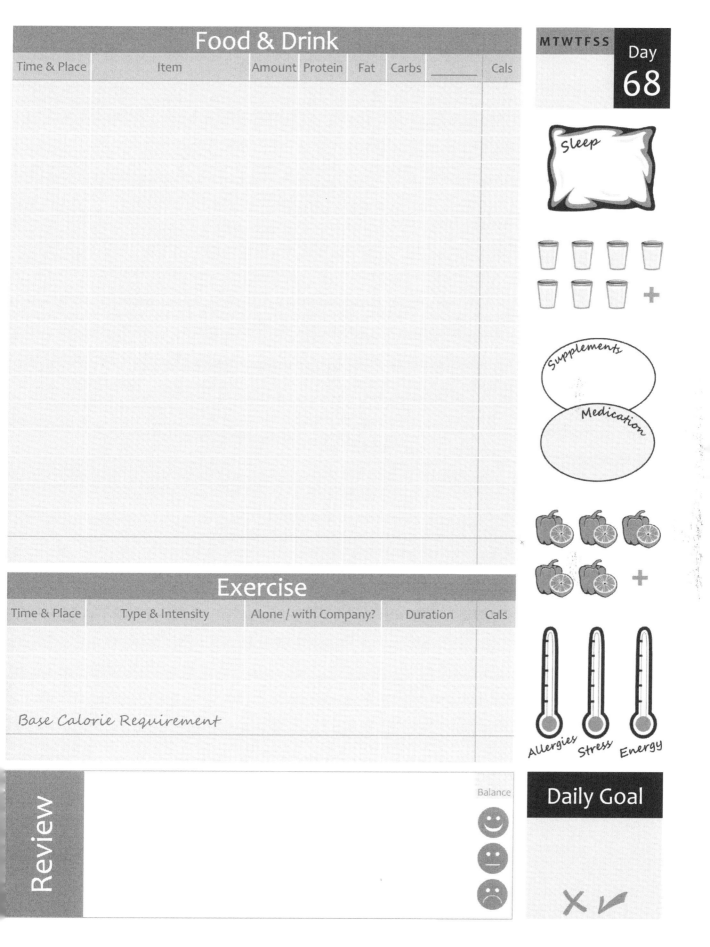

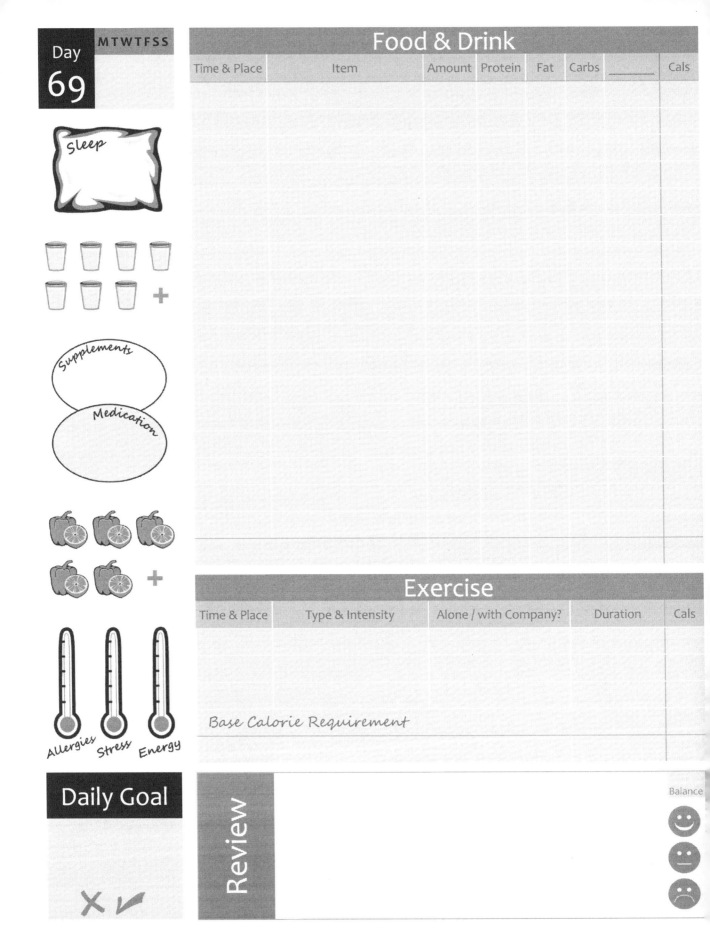

Sleep

Supplements

Medication

Allergies Stress Energy

Daily Goal

X ✔

Food & Drink

Time & Place	Item	Amount	Protein	Fat	Carbs		Cals

Exercise

Time & Place	Type & Intensity	Alone / with Company?	Duration	Cals

Base Calorie Requirement

Review

Balance

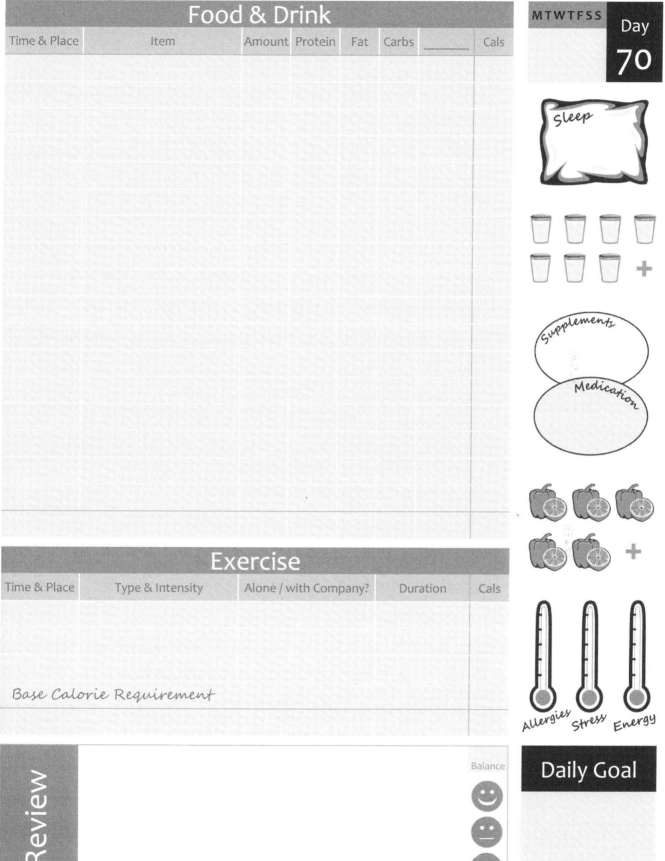

Food & Drink

Time & Place	Item	Amount	Protein	Fat	Carbs	_____	Cals

Sleep

Supplements

Medication

Exercise

Time & Place	Type & Intensity	Alone / with Company?	Duration	Cals

Base Calorie Requirement

Allergies   Stress   Energy

Review

Balance

Daily Goal

X ✔

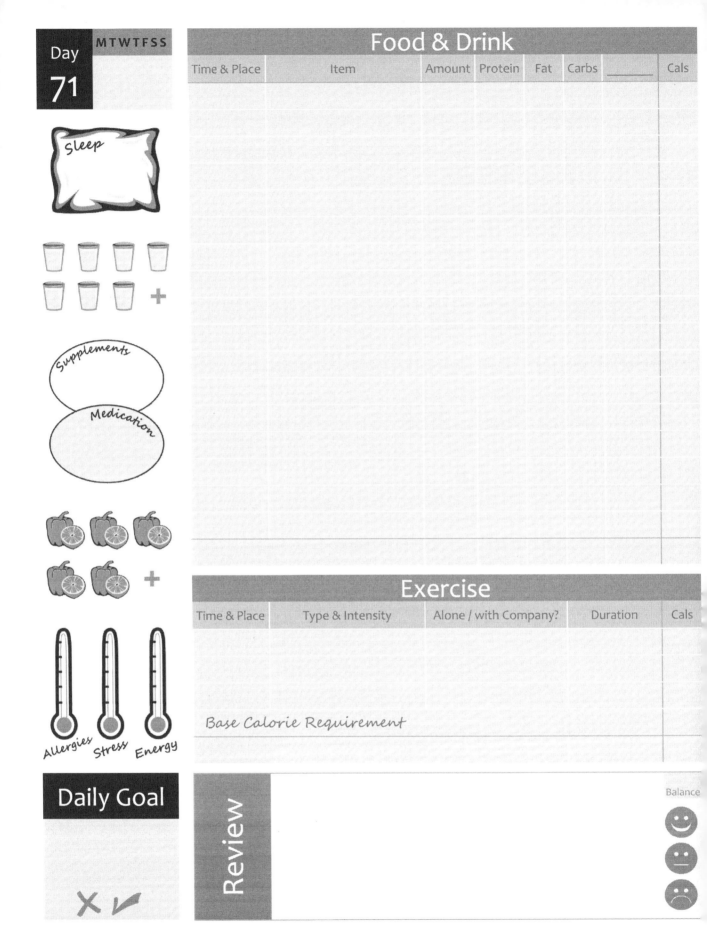

Sleep

Supplements

Medication

Allergies Stress Energy

Daily Goal

X ✔

Food & Drink

Time & Place	Item	Amount	Protein	Fat	Carbs	_____	Cals

Exercise

Time & Place	Type & Intensity	Alone / with Company?	Duration	Cals
Base Calorie Requirement				

Review

Balance

😊

😐

☹️

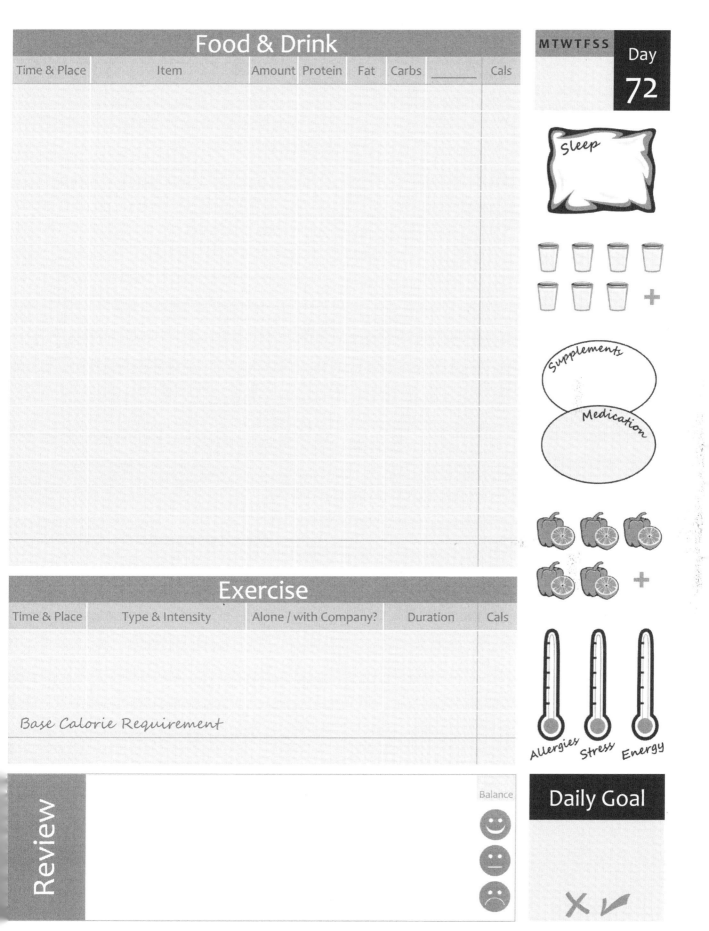

Food & Drink

Time & Place	Item	Amount	Protein	Fat	Carbs	_____	Cals

Sleep

Supplements

Medication

Exercise

Time & Place	Type & Intensity	Alone / with Company?	Duration	Cals
Base Calorie Requirement				

Allergies   Stress   Energy

Review

Balance

Daily Goal

X ✔

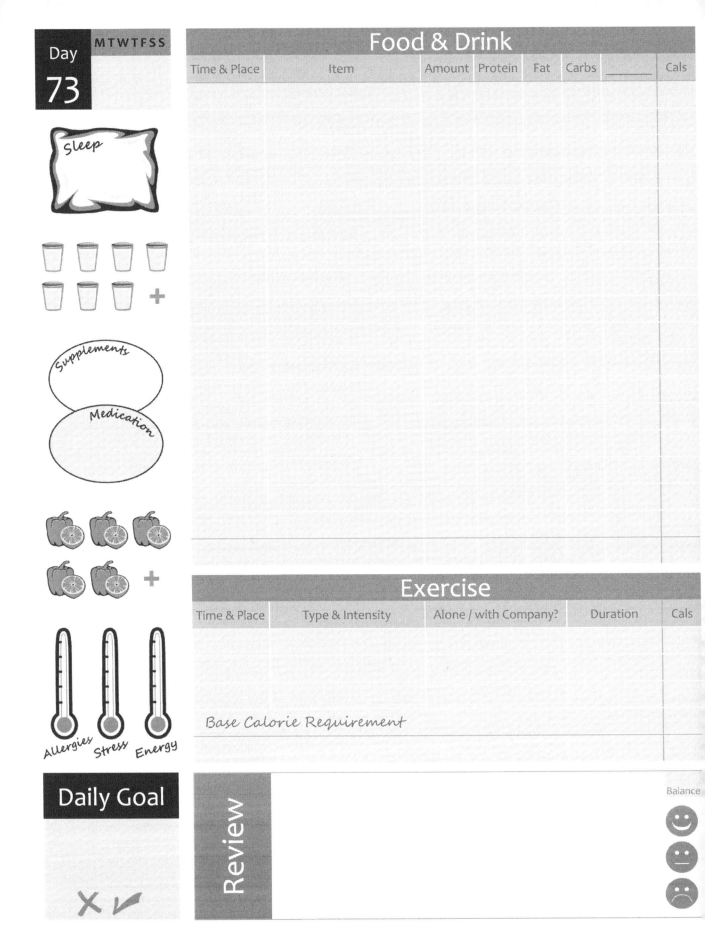

Day
73

MTWTFSS

Sleep

Supplements

Medication

Allergies   Stress   Energy

Daily Goal

X ✔

Food & Drink

Time & Place	Item	Amount	Protein	Fat	Carbs	_____	Cals

Exercise

Time & Place	Type & Intensity	Alone / with Company?	Duration	Cals
Base Calorie Requirement				

Review

Balance

Food & Drink

Time & Place	Item	Amount	Protein	Fat	Carbs	_____	Cals

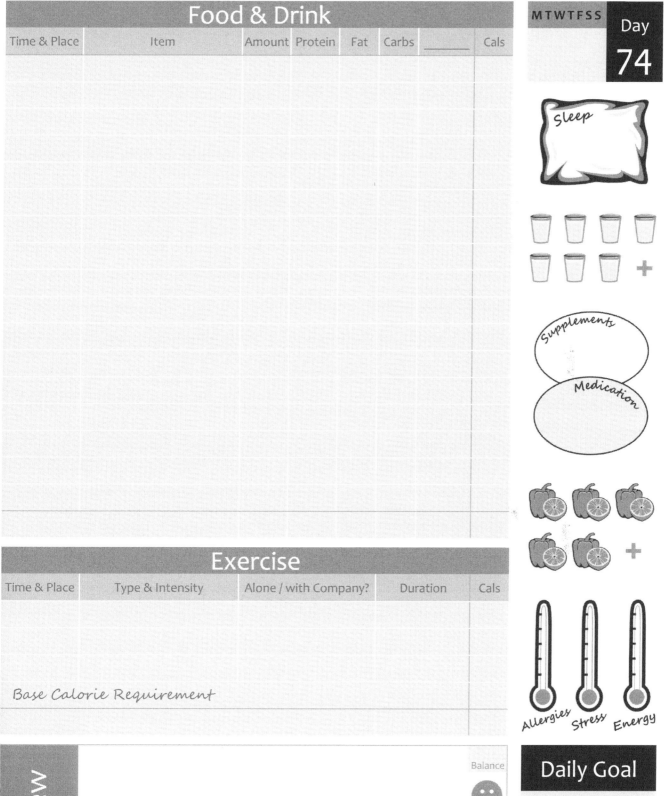

Sleep

Supplements

Medication

Exercise

Time & Place	Type & Intensity	Alone / with Company?	Duration	Cals
Base Calorie Requirement				

Allergies   Stress   Energy

Review

Balance

Daily Goal

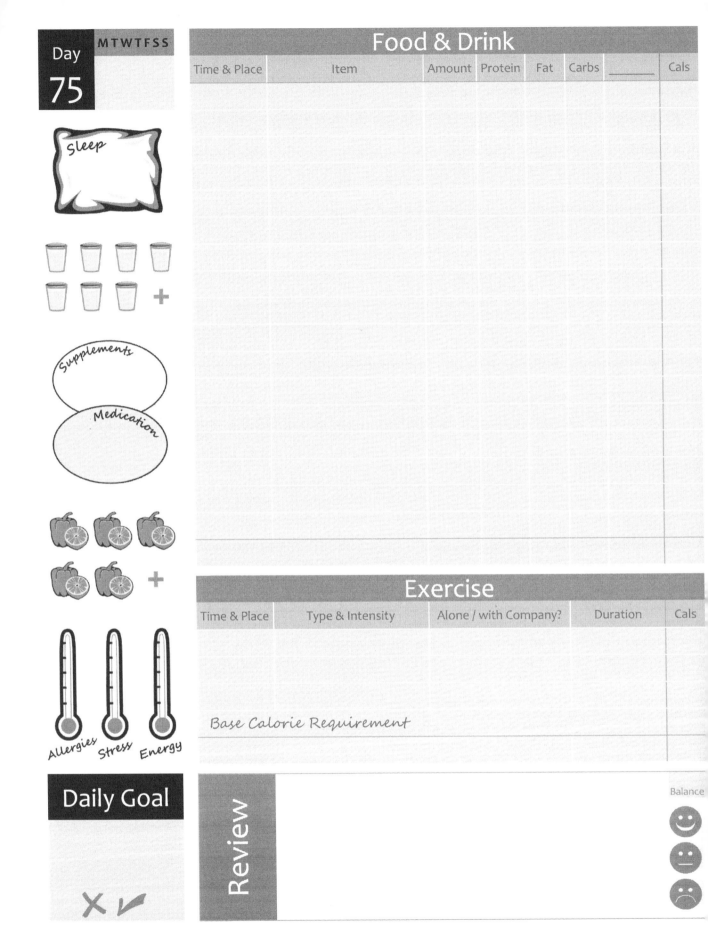

Day 75

MTWTFSS

Sleep

Supplements

Medication

Allergies Stress Energy

Daily Goal

X ✔

Food & Drink

Time & Place	Item	Amount	Protein	Fat	Carbs	_____	Cals

Exercise

Time & Place	Type & Intensity	Alone / with Company?	Duration	Cals

Base Calorie Requirement

Review

Balance

Food & Drink

Time & Place	Item	Amount	Protein	Fat	Carbs	_____	Cals

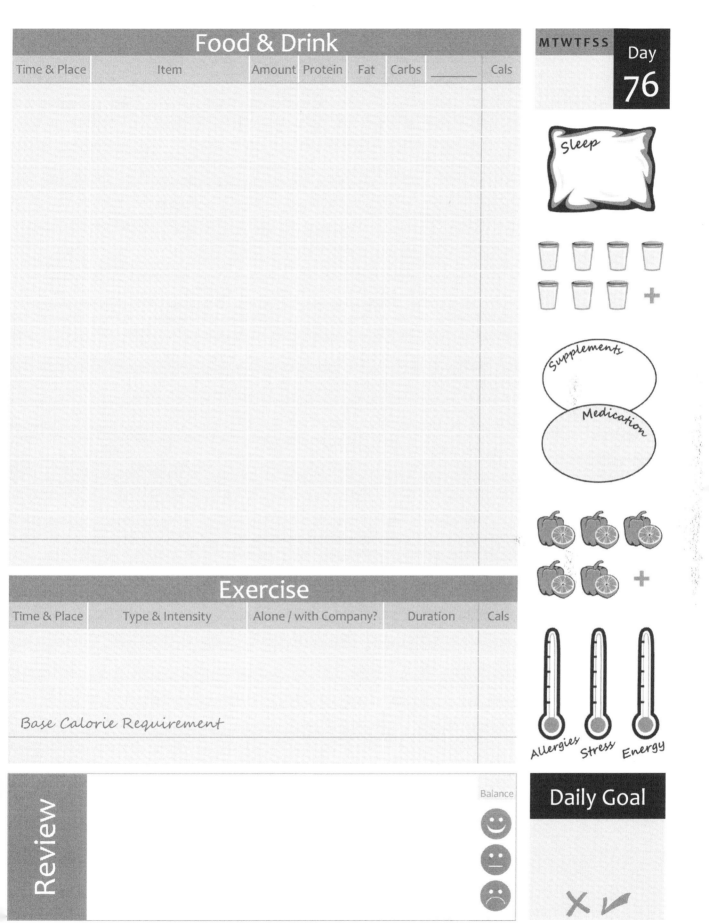

Sleep

Supplements

Medication

Exercise

Time & Place	Type & Intensity	Alone / with Company?	Duration	Cals
Base Calorie Requirement				

Allergies Stress Energy

Review

Balance

Daily Goal

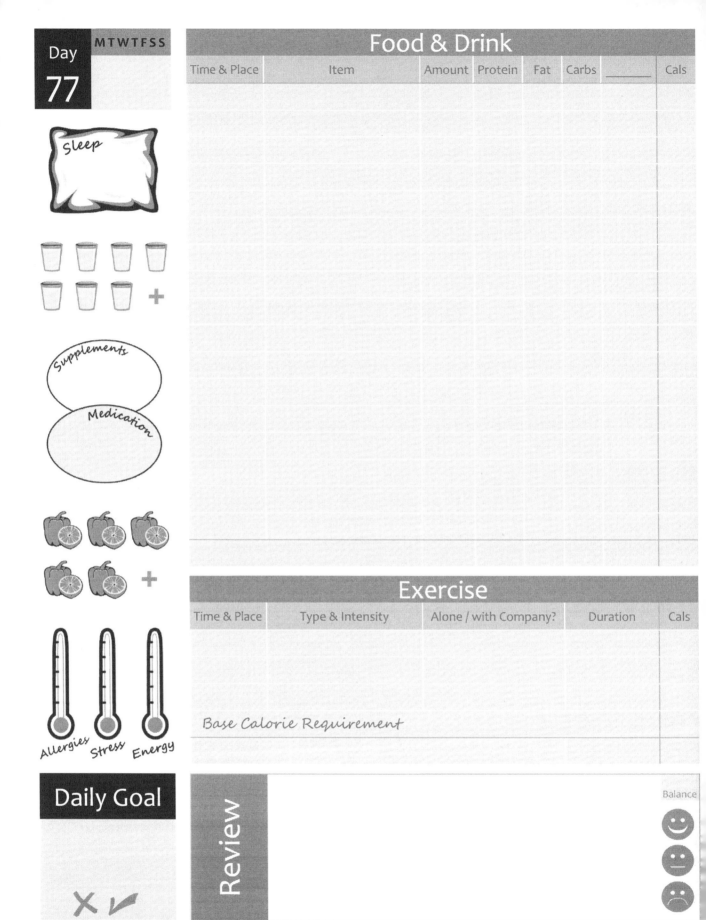

Day 77

MTWTFSS

Sleep

Supplements

Medication

Allergies Stress Energy

Daily Goal

X ✔

Food & Drink

Time & Place	Item	Amount	Protein	Fat	Carbs	_____	Cals

Exercise

Time & Place	Type & Intensity	Alone / with Company?	Duration	Cals
Base Calorie Requirement				

Review

Balance

Food & Drink

Time & Place	Item	Amount	Protein	Fat	Carbs	_____	Cals

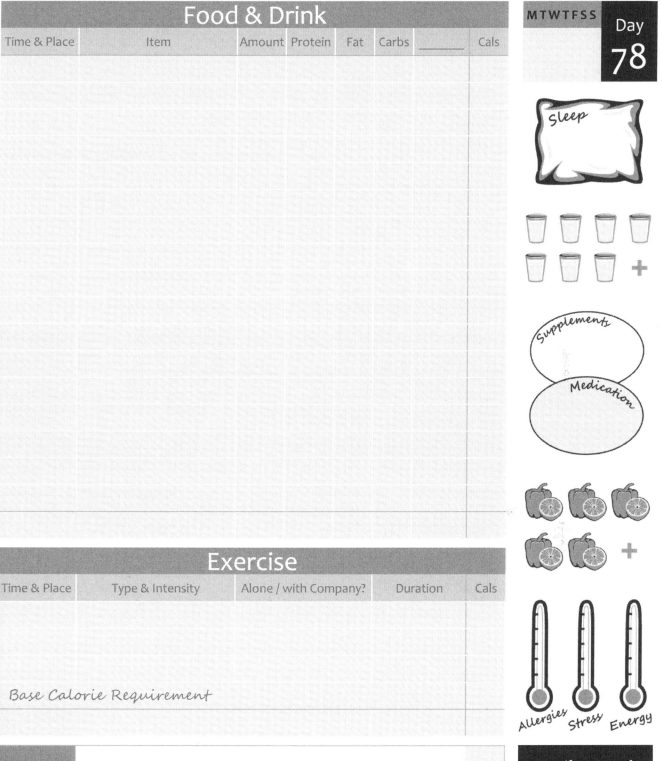

Sleep

Supplements

Medication

Exercise

Time & Place	Type & Intensity	Alone / with Company?	Duration	Cals
Base Calorie Requirement				

Allergies Stress Energy

Review

Balance

Daily Goal

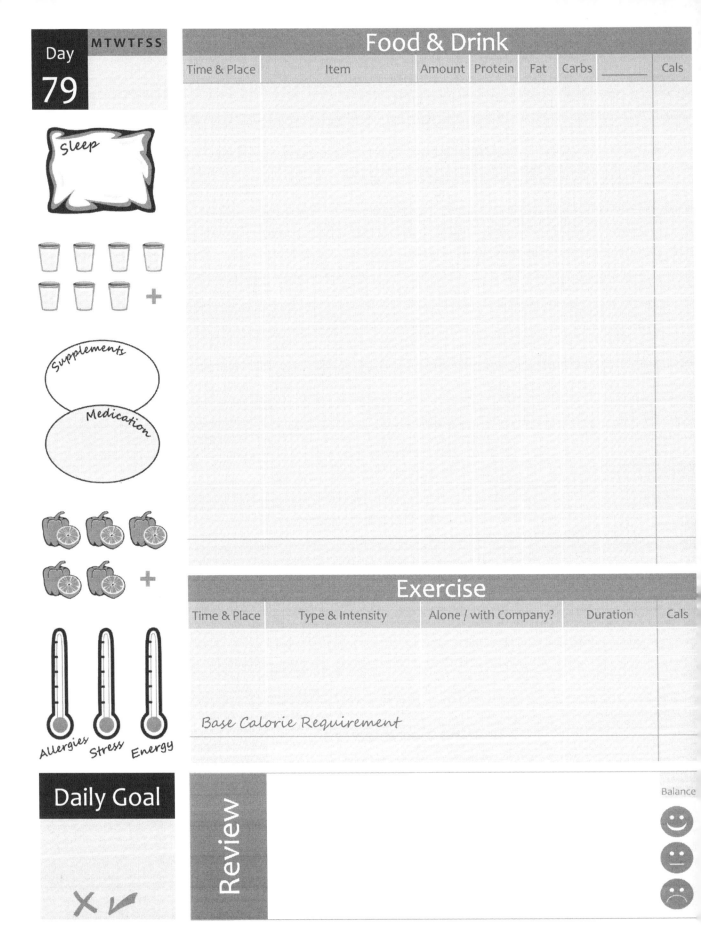

Food & Drink

Time & Place	Item	Amount	Protein	Fat	Carbs	_____	Cals

Sleep

Supplements

Medication

Allergies   Stress   Energy

Exercise

Time & Place	Type & Intensity	Alone / with Company?	Duration	Cals

Base Calorie Requirement

Daily Goal

X ✔

Review

Balance

Food & Drink

Time & Place	Item	Amount	Protein	Fat	Carbs	_____	Cals

Exercise

Time & Place	Type & Intensity	Alone / with Company?	Duration	Cals
Base Calorie Requirement				

Sleep

Supplements

Medication

Allergies   Stress   Energy

Review

Balance

Daily Goal

X ✔

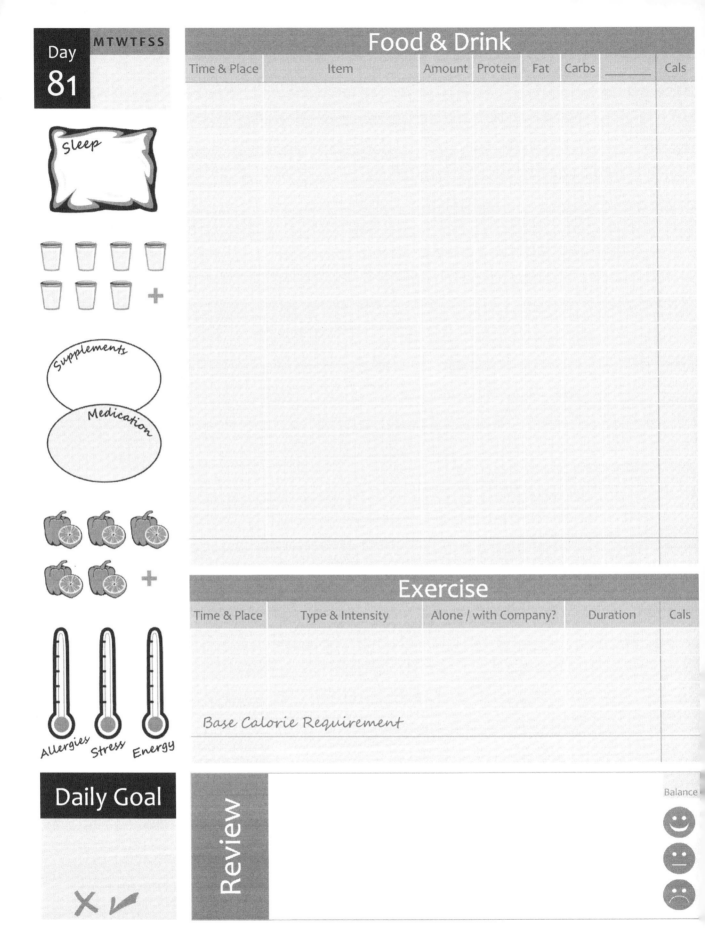

Day 81

MTWTFSS

Sleep

Supplements

Medication

Allergies Stress Energy

Daily Goal

X ✔

Food & Drink

Time & Place	Item	Amount	Protein	Fat	Carbs	____	Cals

Exercise

Time & Place	Type & Intensity	Alone / with Company?	Duration	Cals

Base Calorie Requirement

Review

Balance

Food & Drink

Time & Place	Item	Amount	Protein	Fat	Carbs	_____	Cals

Sleep

Supplements

Medication

Exercise

Time & Place	Type & Intensity	Alone / with Company?	Duration	Cals

Base Calorie Requirement

Allergies Stress Energy

Review

Balance

Daily Goal

X ✔

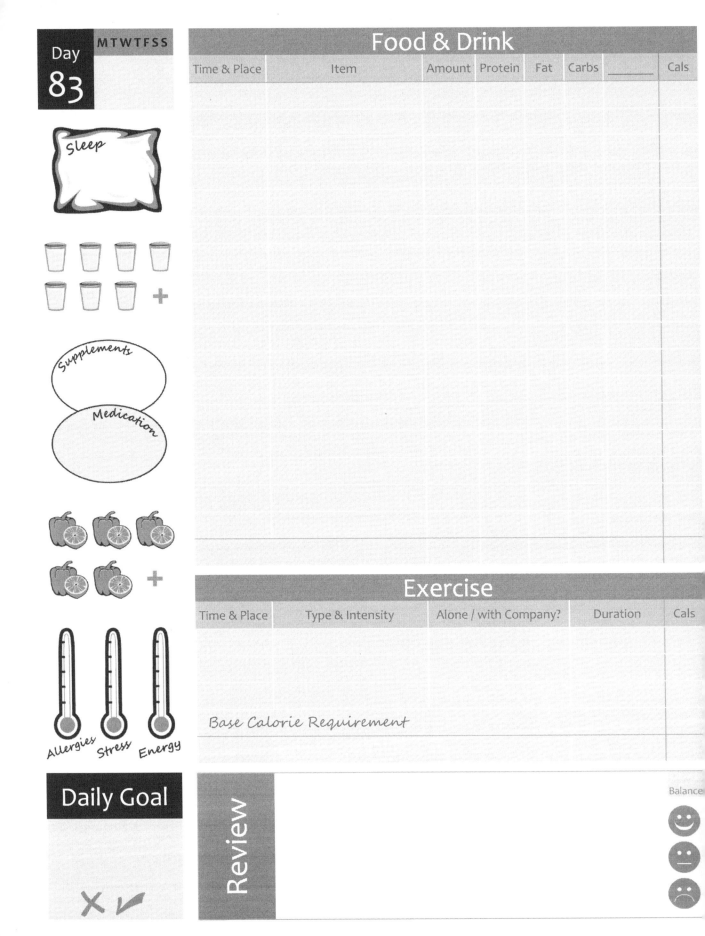

Sleep

Supplements

Medication

Allergies   Stress   Energy

Daily Goal

X ✔

Food & Drink

Time & Place	Item	Amount	Protein	Fat	Carbs	_____	Cals

Exercise

Time & Place	Type & Intensity	Alone / with Company?	Duration	Cals

Base Calorie Requirement

Review

Balance

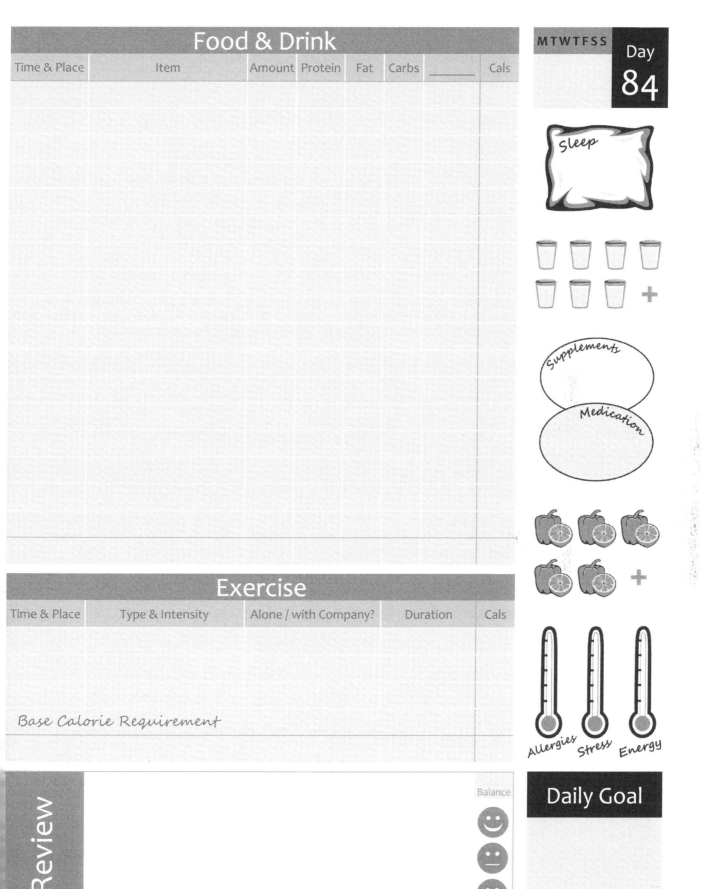

Food & Drink

Time & Place	Item	Amount	Protein	Fat	Carbs	_____	Cals

Sleep

Supplements

Medication

Exercise

Time & Place	Type & Intensity	Alone / with Company?	Duration	Cals

Base Calorie Requirement

Allergies   Stress   Energy

Review

Balance

Daily Goal

X ✔

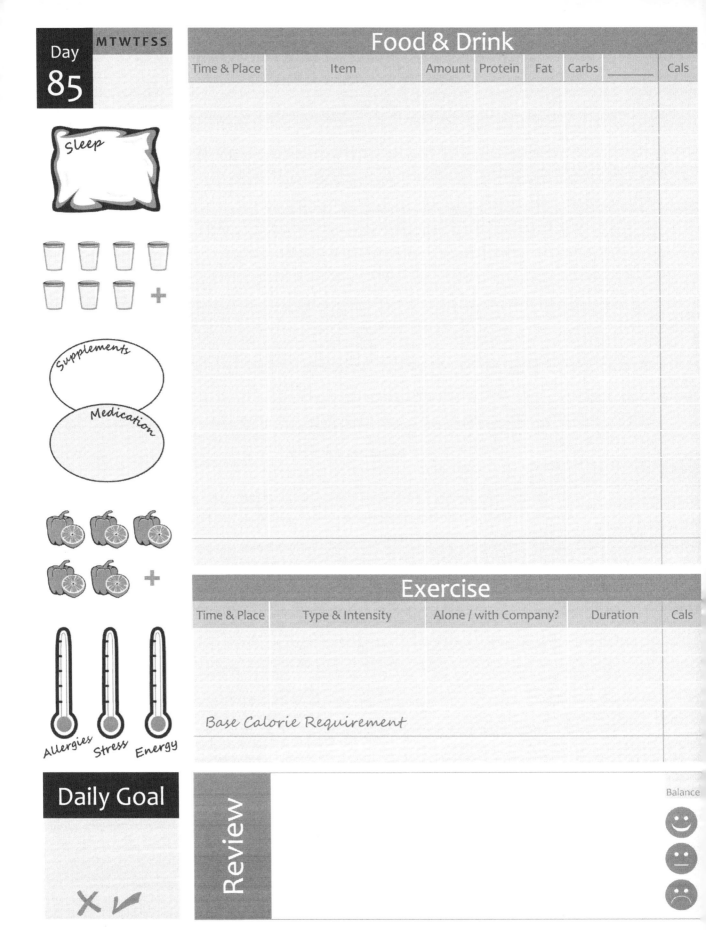

Day	M T W T F S S
85	

Sleep

Supplements

Medication

Allergies Stress Energy

Daily Goal

✗ ✓

Food & Drink

Time & Place	Item	Amount	Protein	Fat	Carbs	_____	Cals

Exercise

Time & Place	Type & Intensity	Alone / with Company?	Duration	Cals
Base Calorie Requirement				

Review

Balance

Food & Drink

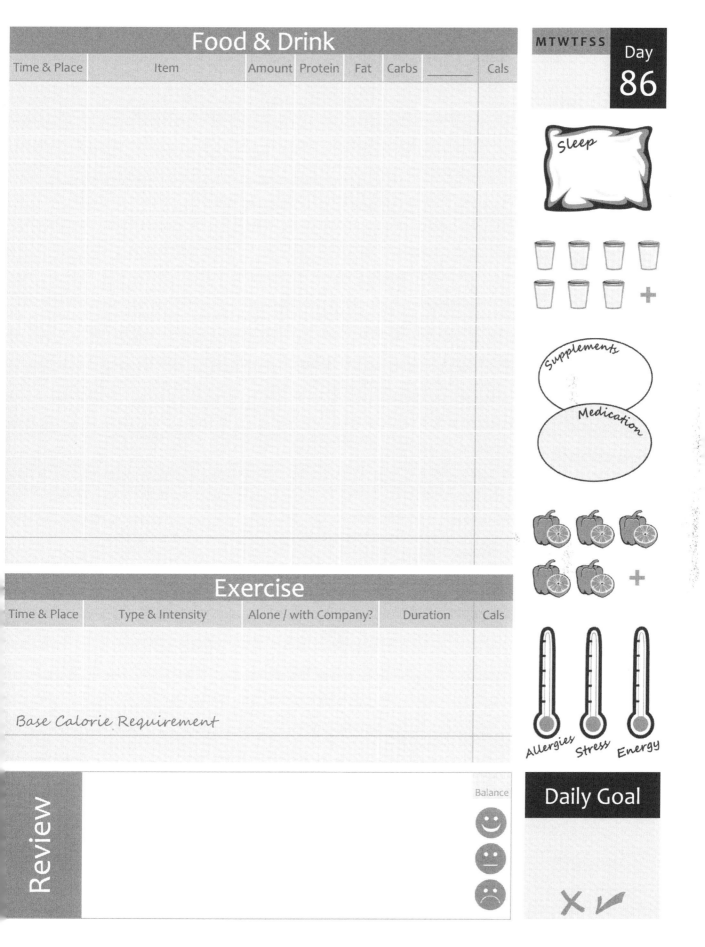

Time & Place	Item	Amount	Protein	Fat	Carbs	_____	Cals

MTWTFSS

Day
86

Sleep

Supplements

Medication

Exercise

Time & Place	Type & Intensity	Alone / with Company?	Duration	Cals

Base Calorie Requirement

Allergies Stress Energy

Review

Balance

Daily Goal

✗ ✔

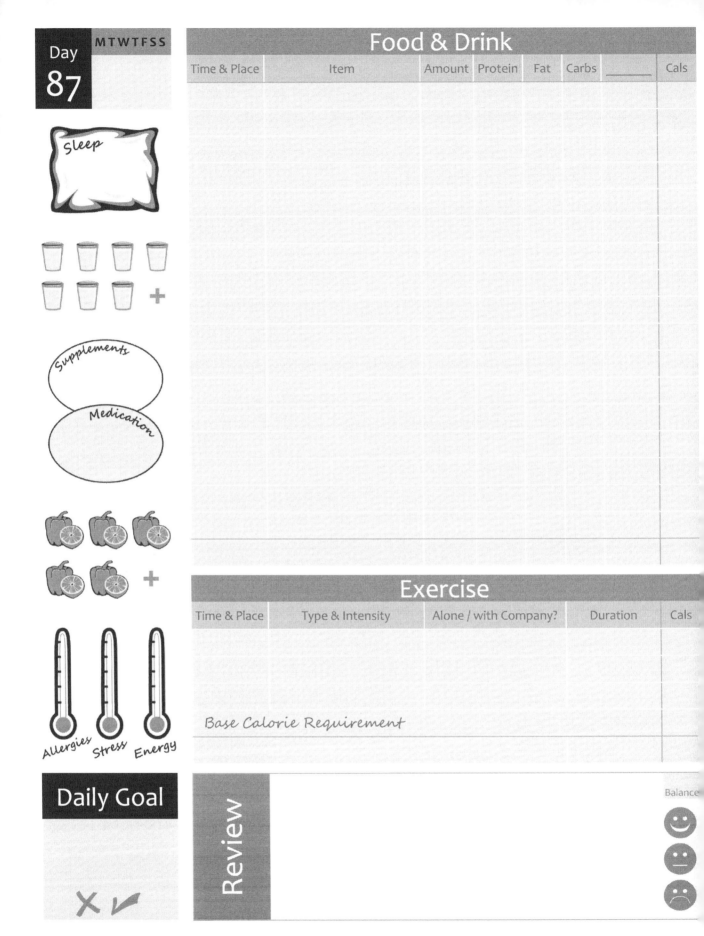

Sleep

Supplements

Medication

Allergies   Stress   Energy

Daily Goal

X ✔

Food & Drink

Time & Place	Item	Amount	Protein	Fat	Carbs	_____	Cals

Exercise

Time & Place	Type & Intensity	Alone / with Company?	Duration	Cals
Base Calorie Requirement				

Review

Balance

Food & Drink

Time & Place	Item	Amount	Protein	Fat	Carbs	_____	Cals

Sleep

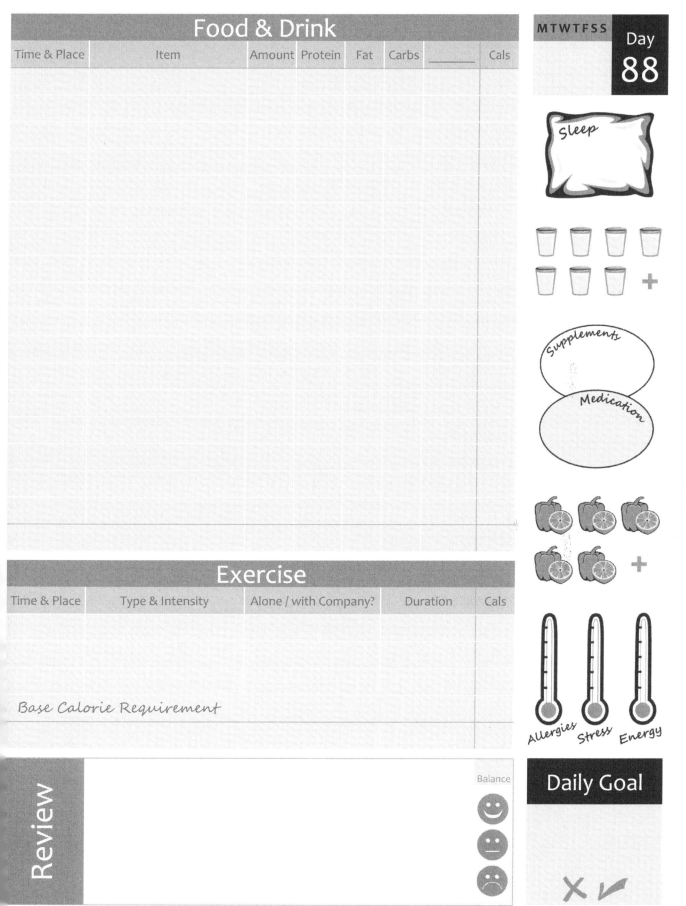

Supplements

Medication

Exercise

Time & Place	Type & Intensity	Alone / with Company?	Duration	Cals

Base Calorie Requirement

Allergies   Stress   Energy

Review

Balance

Daily Goal

X ✔

Sleep

Supplements

Medication

Allergies Stress Energy

Daily Goal

X ✓

Food & Drink

Time & Place	Item	Amount	Protein	Fat	Carbs	____	Cals

Exercise

Time & Place	Type & Intensity	Alone / with Company?	Duration	Cals

Base Calorie Requirement

Review

Balance

Food & Drink

Time & Place	Item	Amount	Protein	Fat	Carbs	_____	Cals

Sleep

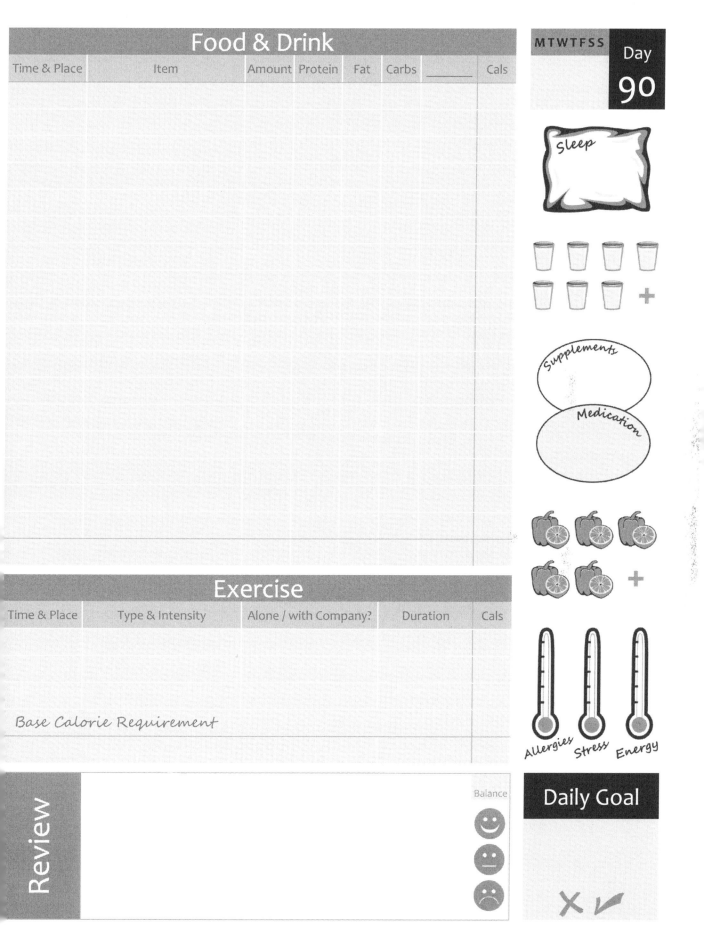

Supplements

Medication

Exercise

Time & Place	Type & Intensity	Alone / with Company?	Duration	Cals
Base Calorie Requirement				

Allergies　Stress　Energy

Review

Balance

Daily Goal

X ✔

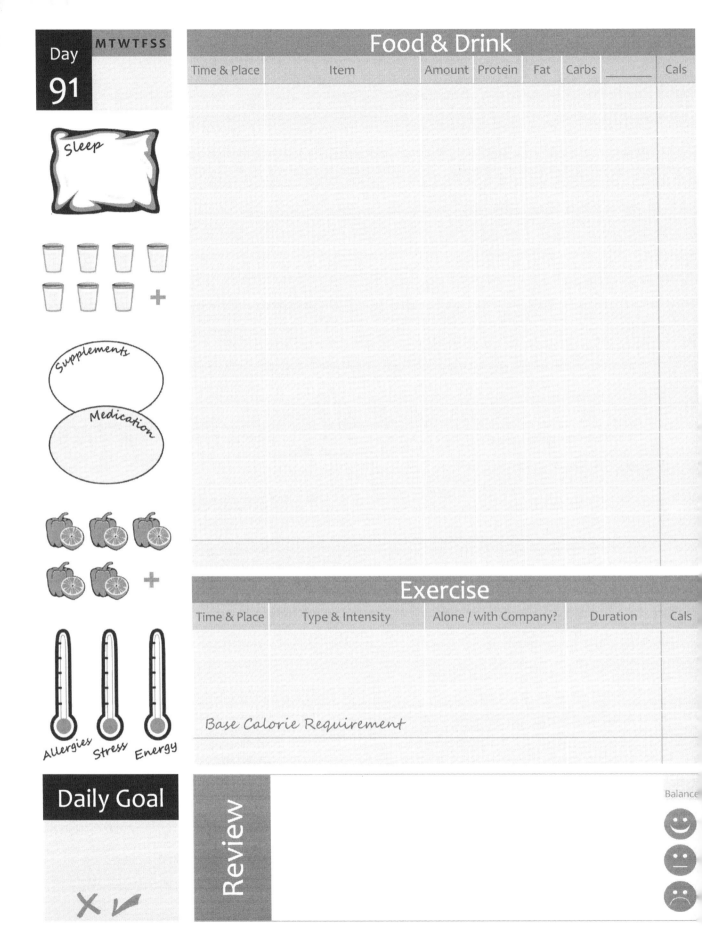

Day
91

MTWTFSS

Sleep

Supplements

Medication

Allergies Stress Energy

Daily Goal

X ✔

Food & Drink

Time & Place	Item	Amount	Protein	Fat	Carbs	_____	Cals

Exercise

Time & Place	Type & Intensity	Alone / with Company?	Duration	Cals

Base Calorie Requirement

Review

Balance

Food & Drink

Time & Place	Item	Amount	Protein	Fat	Carbs	_____	Cals

Sleep

Supplements

Medication

Exercise

Time & Place	Type & Intensity	Alone / with Company?	Duration	Cals
Base Calorie Requirement				

Allergies Stress Energy

Review

Balance

Daily Goal

X ✔

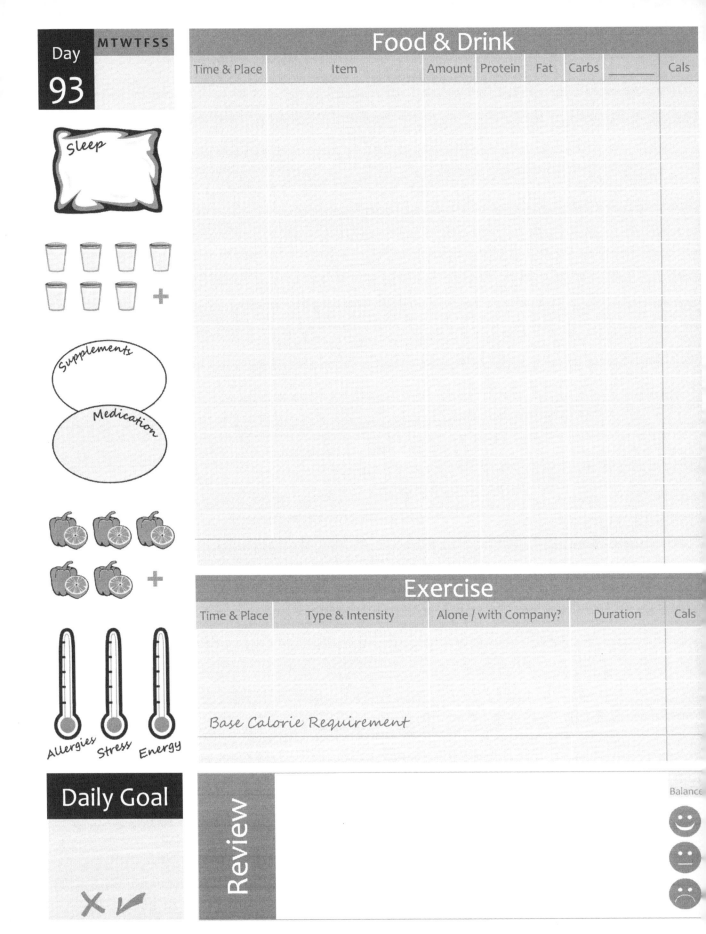

Day 93

MTWTFSS

Sleep

Supplements

Medication

Allergies Stress Energy

Daily Goal

X ✓

Food & Drink

Time & Place	Item	Amount	Protein	Fat	Carbs	_____	Cals

Exercise

Time & Place	Type & Intensity	Alone / with Company?	Duration	Cals

Base Calorie Requirement

Review

Balance

Food & Drink

Time & Place	Item	Amount	Protein	Fat	Carbs	_____	Cals

Sleep

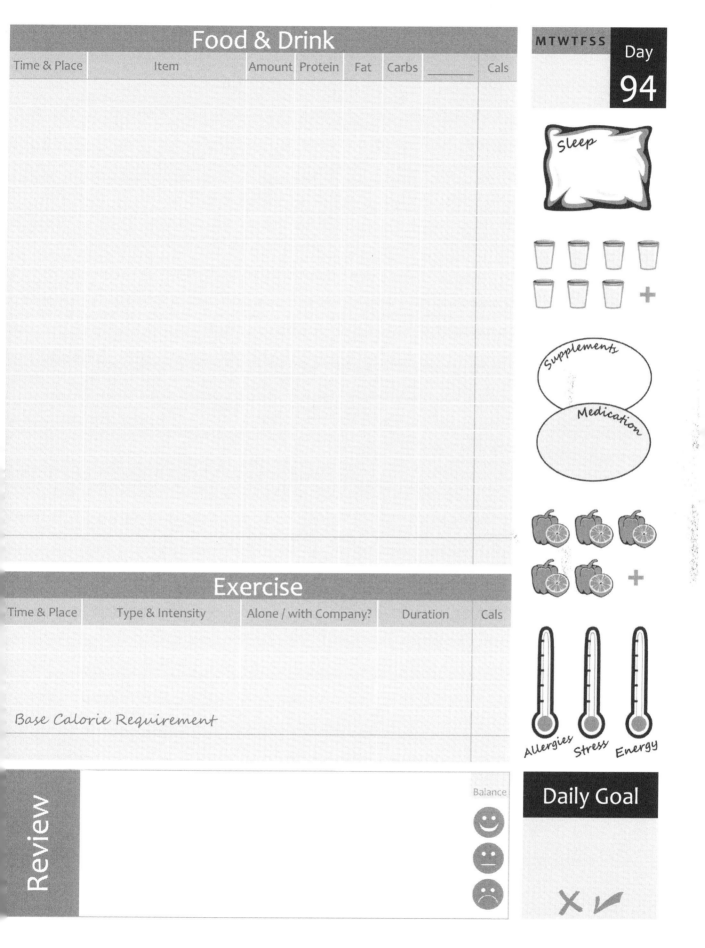

Supplements

Medication

Exercise

Time & Place	Type & Intensity	Alone / with Company?	Duration	Cals

Base Calorie Requirement

Allergies   Stress   Energy

Review

Balance

Daily Goal

X ✔

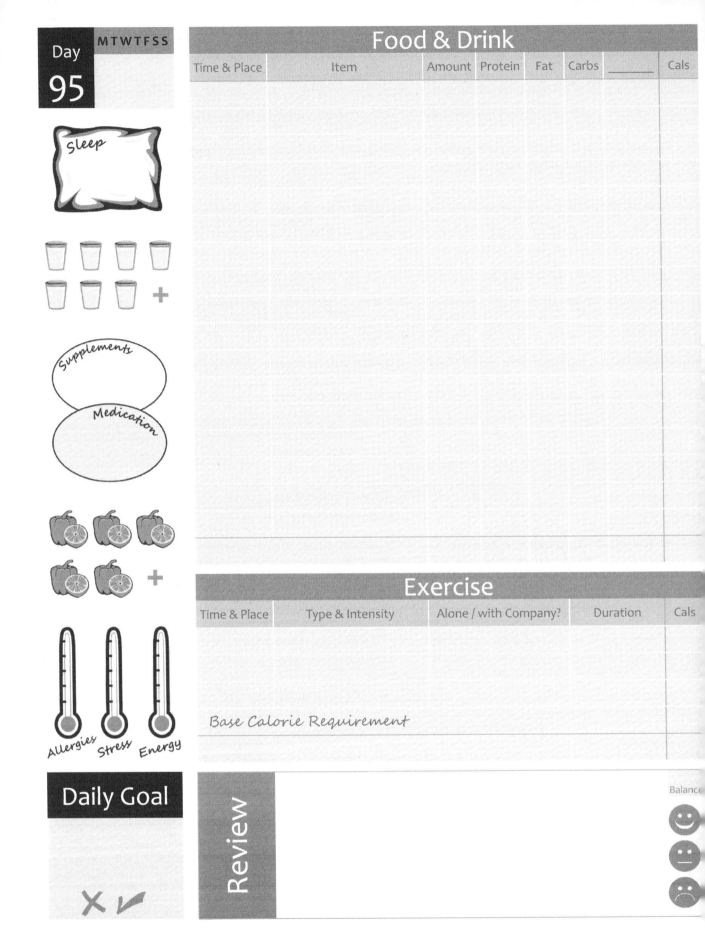

Day 95

MTWTFSS

Sleep

Supplements

Medication

Allergies Stress Energy

Daily Goal

X ✔

Food & Drink

Time & Place	Item	Amount	Protein	Fat	Carbs	_____	Cals

Exercise

Time & Place	Type & Intensity	Alone / with Company?	Duration	Cals

Base Calorie Requirement

Review

Balance

Food & Drink

Time & Place	Item	Amount	Protein	Fat	Carbs	_____	Cals

Sleep

Supplements

Medication

+

+

Allergies Stress Energy

Exercise

Time & Place	Type & Intensity	Alone / with Company?	Duration	Cals

Base Calorie Requirement

Review

Balance

Daily Goal

X ✔

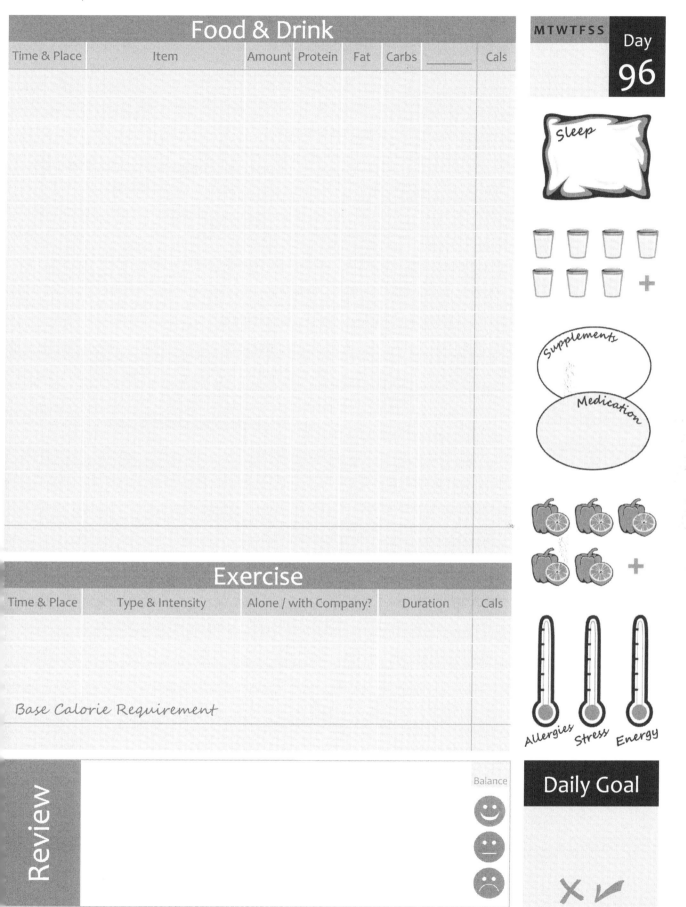

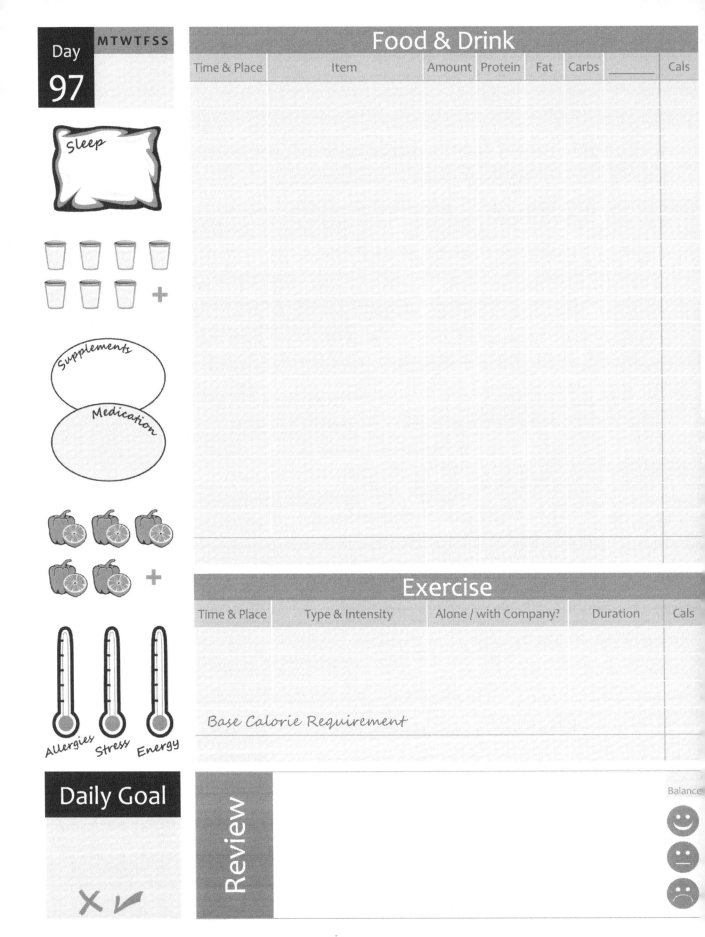

Day
97

MTWTFSS

Sleep

Supplements

Medication

Allergies Stress Energy

Daily Goal

X ✔

Food & Drink

Time & Place	Item	Amount	Protein	Fat	Carbs	_____	Cals

Exercise

Time & Place	Type & Intensity	Alone / with Company?	Duration	Cals
Base Calorie Requirement				

Review

Balance

Food & Drink

Time & Place	Item	Amount	Protein	Fat	Carbs	_____	Cals

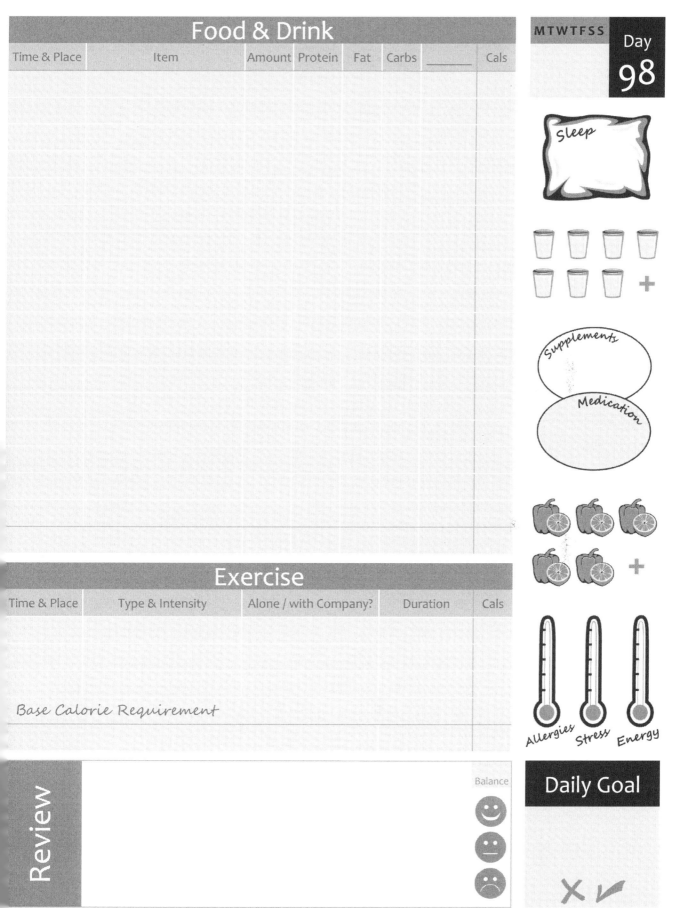

Sleep

Supplements

Medication

Exercise

Time & Place	Type & Intensity	Alone / with Company?	Duration	Cals
Base Calorie Requirement				

Allergies   Stress   Energy

Review

Balance

Daily Goal

X ✔

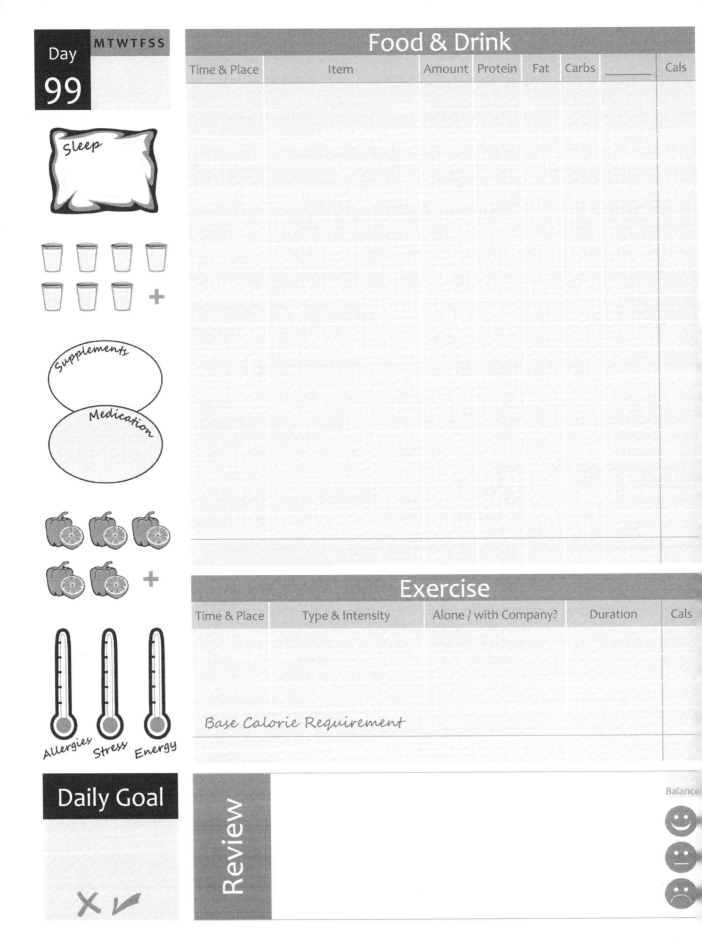

Day 99

MTWTFSS

Sleep

Supplements

Medication

Allergies Stress Energy

Daily Goal

X ✔

Food & Drink

Time & Place	Item	Amount	Protein	Fat	Carbs	_____	Cals

Exercise

Time & Place	Type & Intensity	Alone / with Company?	Duration	Cals
Base Calorie Requirement				

Review

Balance

Food & Drink

Time & Place	Item	Amount	Protein	Fat	Carbs	_____	Cals

Sleep

Supplements

Medication

Exercise

Time & Place	Type & Intensity	Alone / with Company?	Duration	Cals

Base Calorie Requirement

Allergies Stress Energy

Review

Balance

Daily Goal

X ✔

Calorie Expenditure

Base Calorie Requirements when Sedentary

Age	Men	Women
16-18	2400	1800
19-20	2600	2000
21-25	2400	2000
26-40	2400	1800
41-50	2200	1800
51-60	2200	1600
61+	2000	1600

Calorie Expenditure during Exercise (per minute)

Activity	Body weight			
	56kg / 124lb	62kg / 137lb	68kg / 150lb	74kg / 163lb
Badminton	5.4	6.0	6.6	7.2
Basketball	7.7	8.6	9.4	10.2
Canoeing - leisurely	2.5	2.7	3.0	3.3
Climbing	6.8	7.5	8.2	9.0
Circuits / Aerobics – medium	5.8	6.4	7.0	7.6
Circuits / Aerobics - intense	7.5	8.3	9.2	10.0
Cycling – leisure	5.6	6.2	6.8	7.4
Cycling – racing	9.5	10.5	11.5	12.5
Hockey	7.5	8.3	9.2	10.0
Golf	4.8	5.3	5.8	6.3
Gymnastics	3.7	4.1	4.5	4.9
Judo	10.9	12.1	13.3	14.4
Running – 11.5 min/mile	7.6	8.4	9.2	10.0
Running – 8 min/mile	11.9	13.1	14.2	15.4
Skiing – cross country	6.7	7.4	8.1	8.8
Skiing – down hill	5.7	6.5	7.1	7.7
Soccer	7.4	8.2	9.0	9.8
Standing up	2.1	2.3	2.4	2.7
Squash	11.9	13.1	14.4	15.7
Swimming – breast stroke	9.1	10.0	11.0	12.0
Swimming – fast crawl	8.7	9.7	10.6	11.5
Swimming – slow crawl	7.2	7.9	8.7	9.5
Tennis - singles	6.1	6.8	7.4	8.1
Walking at medium pace	4.6	5.1	5.3	6.0

Personal Nutrition Charts

Use these tables to store data on meals or foods that you regularly eat, for quick reference.

Item	Amount	Protein	Fat	Carbs		Calories

Item	Amount	Protein	Fat	Carbs		Calories

Item	Amount	Protein	Fat	Carbs		Calories

Item	Amount	Protein	Fat	Carbs		Calories

Item	Amount	Protein	Fat	Carbs		Calories

Item	Amount	Protein	Fat	Carbs		Calories

Item	Amount	Protein	Fat	Carbs		Calories

Item	Amount	Protein	Fat	Carbs		Calories

Item	Amount	Protein	Fat	Carbs		Calories

Statistics Tracker

Day No. or Date	Weight	Waist	Cholesterol	Blood Pressure	Morning Heart Rate	Body Fat			Daily Goals going Forwards

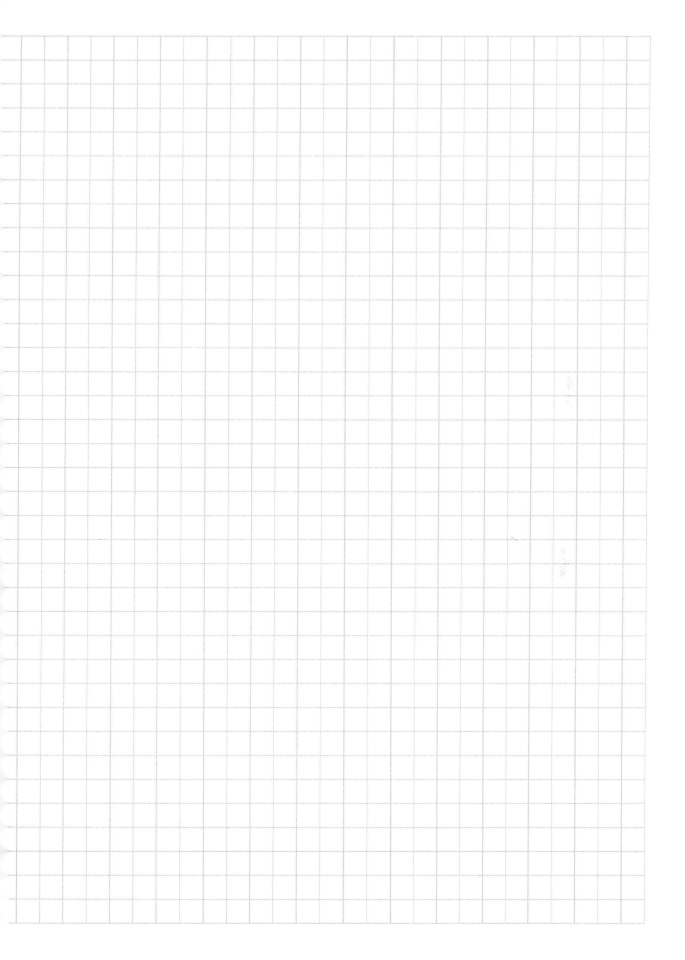

Notes

Printed in Great Britain
by Amazon

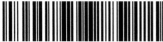